# Leaders in Plastic Surgery

# Leaders in Plastic Surgery

The Dingman–Grabb Era 1946–1986
at the University of Michigan and
Saint Joseph Mercy Hospital
in Ann Arbor, Michigan

**By Robert M. Oneal, MD,
and Lauralee A. Lutz**

Copyright © 2017 by the Regents of the University of Michigan
Some rights reserved

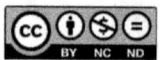

This work is licensed under the Creative Commons Attribution-NonCommercial-NoDerivatives 4.0 International License. To view a copy of this license, visit http://creativecommons.org/licenses/by-nc-nd/4.0/ or send a letter to Creative Commons, PO Box 1866, Mountain View, California, 94042, USA.

Published in the United States of America by
Michigan Publishing
Manufactured in the United States of America

DOI: http://dx.doi.org/10.3998/maize.mpub9470414

ISBN 978-1-60785-385-5 (paper)
ISBN 978-1-60785-386-2 (e-book)

An imprint of Michigan Publishing, Maize Books serves the publishing needs of the University of Michigan community by making high-quality scholarship widely available in print and online. It represents a new model for authors seeking to share their work within and beyond the academy, offering streamlined selection, production, and distribution processes. Maize Books is intended as a complement to more formal modes of publication in a wide range of disciplinary areas.

http://www.maizebooks.org

# Dedicated to

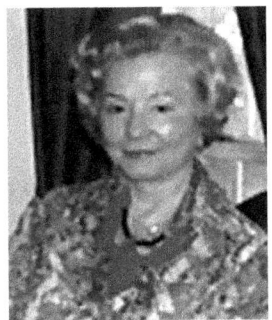
Thelma Muir Dingman

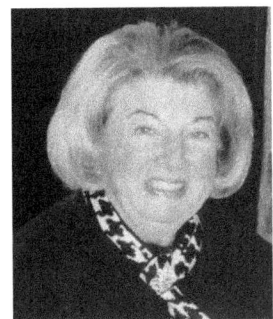
Cozette Tweedie Grabb

Thelma Muir Dingman (wife of Reed O. Dingman) and Cozette Tweedie Grabb (wife of William C. Grabb), for their enduring love, support, and inspiration, as well as their generous hospitality, all contributing so much to the growth and future success of plastic surgery in Ann Arbor and beyond.

# Image Credits

**Courtesy of Bentley Historical Library, University of Michigan:**

Photo 2: #HS12895, UM Dental School
Photo 13: #BL004572, UM Medical School
Photo 18: #BL004572, UM Medical School
Photo 20: #HS6083, UM School of Art and Design

**Courtesy of Regents of the University of Michigan:**

Photos 4, 6, 10, 14, 16, 24, 28, 30, 34, 37, 38, 39, 45, 50, 56, 70

**We thank the following people for their gracious permission to use their images:**

*Robert Gilman:* Photos 19, 23, 25, 31, 33, 40, 48, 49, 53
*David Dingman:* Photos 1, 3, 12, 42, 54, 58, 59, A5, A18
*Robert Oneal:* Photos 9, 11, 41, 48, 52, 66, A8, A9, A10, A12, A19
*Terry Cromwell:* Photo of Thelma Muir Dingman (Dedication)
    Photos 8, 15, 64, 65
*Cozette Grabb:* Photos 17, 46, 67, 68, 69
*Robert Wilensky:* Photos 21, 22, 26, 27
*Sigurdur Thorvalsson:* Photos 29, 35, 36, 57, A16
*Paul Cederna:* Photos 60, 61, 62, 63
*Yvonne Gellise, RSM:* Photos 5, 7, 44
*Chris Hedley:* Photos 32, 43, A6
*Martha McClatchey:* Photo 51
*Anne Chase:* Photo of Cozette Tweedie Grabb (Dedication)
*Richard Sarns:* Photo 55
*Lauralee A. Lutz:* Photos 24, A6, A7, A9, A11, A13, A14, A15, A17
*James C. Norris:* Photo A6
*Harvey Weiss*: Photo 62

# Contents

Foreword ix
Preface xi
Acknowledgments xiii

**CHAPTER ONE**
Early Influences on the Development
of Plastic Surgery in Ann Arbor, Michigan    1

**CHAPTER TWO**
Origin of Plastic Surgery Residency Training
at Saint Joseph Mercy Hospital in Ann Arbor    6

**CHAPTER THREE**
Creation of the Section of Plastic Surgery in
the University of Michigan Department of Surgery    11

**CHAPTER FOUR**
Transitions in the Section of Plastic Surgery    23

**CHAPTER FIVE**
Early Clinical Rotations and Teaching Conferences    39

**CHAPTER SIX**
Research Activities and the
F. Roland Sargent Research Laboratory    53

**CHAPTER SEVEN**
Clinical Research, Clinical Procedures,
New Techniques—1946–86    66

## CHAPTER EIGHT
Plastic Surgery Extending beyond Ann Arbor
and the University of Michigan 120

## CHAPTER NINE
Reflections and Commentary about Their Ann Arbor
Plastic Surgery Experience by the Authors,
Residents, and Fellows 126

Epilogue 146
Appendix 149
Group Images of Residents 174
References 184
About the Author 194
Index 195

# Foreword

This book is a gift from generation to generation celebrating the remarkable history of plastic surgery at the University of Michigan. Bob Oneal and Lauralee Lutz have given us an expertly crafted and written book describing the growth and development of plastic surgery at the University of Michigan, which began seventy years ago. Through historical facts, events, memories, personal anecdotes, and images, they have captured the essence of our program and given us an opportunity to personally experience the victories and challenges of the pioneers of our program and the leaders of our specialty. From the very early stages of our residency program, the Section of Plastic Surgery, the University of Michigan, has played a pivotal role in defining plastic surgical education in the United States of America and refining the manner in which plastic surgery residents are trained and certified. In clinical terms, whether it was burn patients, cancer survivors, children born with congenital defects, or trauma victims, our plastic surgeons at the University of Michigan have helped to reconstruct lives through their clinical acumen and technical virtuosity. These efforts began in the 1940s and have continued to progress to date. There are many advanced therapeutics, interventions, and surgical approaches we commonly use today that were not even conceivable seventy years ago. It is quite clear that the current developments did not occur over the course of a few years but were rooted in the very foundation of our program in 1946. Our current program stands on the incredible accomplishments of the early pioneers of plastic surgery who developed this foundation. Bob and Lauralee have captured the maturation of our program in their thoughtful, comprehensive, and entertaining book. Not only have the significant developments of the program been expertly documented and the content creatively framed to develop an interesting story, but personal memories, anecdotes, and stories have been sprinkled throughout the book to provide a more personal flavor to the program. It is this combination of notable accomplishments interspersed with personal anecdotes that makes the book so entertaining to read and so valuable as a way to document our rich and illustrious history. You will definitely "feel" what the program was like and understand how our specialty has become what it is after reading this book and reflecting on all of the major contributions of our early leaders from the University of Michigan.

As chief of the Section of Plastic Surgery at the University of Michigan, I could not be happier that Dr. Oneal and Lauralee have written this book. The growth and maturation of our plastic surgery program have paralleled the development of the specialty of plastic surgery. Recognizing these parallels, feeling the excitement as the specialty of plastic surgery matured, and understanding the implications of these developments on the future of our specialty are important for our history and for our future growth. As a graduate of the University of Michigan plastic surgery residency program, I feel privileged to have trained in such a prominent program. I am sure all of our graduates will join me in feeling thankful for this experience. This book very nicely captures the essence of our program during the formative years of our plastic surgery residency training and during the development of our specialty as a whole. I believe anyone interested in the history of medicine and in the development of the specialty of plastic surgery will find this an engaging, interesting, and captivating read. I personally would like to thank Dr. Oneal and Lauralee for this labor of love. I could not be more proud of the program we have at the University of Michigan, Section of Plastic Surgery, and could not be happier about the book that Dr. Oneal and Lauralee have created. Please enjoy reading it as I have.

Paul S. Cederna, MD<br>
Chief, Section of Plastic Surgery<br>
Robert Oneal Professor of Plastic Surgery<br>
Professor, Department of Biomedical Engineering<br>
University of Michigan

# Preface

This book was written to record a history of the Section of Plastic Surgery at the University of Michigan and the career of Reed O. Dingman, DDS, MD. Indeed, the professional life of Dr. Dingman and the creation of a dedicated plastic surgery section were parallel and inseparable. William C. Grabb, MD, one of his early trainees, and subsequently his successor, was an integral part of the University of Michigan program and had a great deal to do with the ongoing development of the training program and the research activities. This book is simply a labor of love and a sincere show of respect for Drs. Reed O. Dingman and William C. Grabb.

I (Bob Oneal) joined the faculty two years after the formation of the Section of Plastic Surgery at the University of Michigan and I am still involved in resident teaching. At the university, people often ask me questions about the persons, procedures, and events from the past history of University of Michigan plastic surgery. Lauralee Lutz offers memories from her vantage point as section executive secretary from 1968 for the remainder of this book's time period. Together, we felt that this history should be recorded before it was forgotten. We hope that this book will be of interest not only to those plastic surgeons who trained in the program during the time frame of the book but also to the many alumni since 1986 and to the generations of trainees to come.

We start with the early days in the development of plastic surgery in Ann Arbor and the foresight of Dr. Dingman who realized the future for training should be connected with the medical school. As the specialty of plastic surgery developed, it began to touch all branches of surgery as well as anatomy and physiology. During this time, Dr. Dingman was an inspiration to two generations of surgeons and stimulated many of us to seek an academic career. His influence continues to date. We especially wanted to record our high regard and affection for Dr. Dingman, our father figure and a special genius who made it all possible. You will read much praise for his private guidance and genuine concern for each trainee. He was our anchor and our sail.

We felt it was important to recall the early development of the faculty and describe the early resident clinical rotations. The early emphasis on plastic surgery research is discussed along with some of the significant projects and ideas during these years. We also felt it important to document the early pioneering clinical work of both Dr. Dingman and Dr. Grabb and how it was shared with the larger plastic surgery community. We also describe, in some detail, the extensive range of clinical activities that the faculty engaged in through the years, some of which have historical significance. Another important aspect to note is that the last quarter of the time frame of this book encompasses the great explosion of plastic surgical knowledge and the development of procedures that transformed the specialty and enabled solutions to conditions thought to be unsolvable. The march of progress continues.

We have also tried to paint a picture of the humanity of this time not only by recounting historical facts and events but also by putting forth personal anecdotes, memories, and impressions of the faculty and many of almost one hundred of the trainees during this time period who took the time out to reflect on their Ann Arbor years. These stories and memories are marvelous contributions.

This book required, and benefited by, inputs from many people and sources, and due credit is given where possible. A heartfelt note of thank you to every contributor who helped us in achieving our goal. We felt it was very important to document all aspects of the foundation of plastic surgery at the University of Michigan and to appreciate the hard work, inspiration, fellowship, and love that went into its development. We did our best to capture this history—so much a forever part of our lives.

Robert M. Oneal MD and Lauralee Lutz

# Acknowledgments

We are extremely grateful for the unfailing help we received from Zibby Oneal during the preparation of this book. Her professional advice about content, rereading, and repeated editing of the entire manuscript during its various stages of preparation was invaluable. Special thanks also to Tiffany Ballard, MD, one of our plastic surgery residents, for help with the initial setup, locating references, and scanning material to be included, as well as for her encouragement, enthusiasm, and determination that were so essential in the early phases of this book. Thanks also to Michael Oneal who added a professional journalist's vision to the introduction of each chapter and elsewhere in the manuscript. We are indebted to Jeanne Mulholland and Debbie Newton, plastic surgery secretaries at the University of Michigan, for the very prompt and competent typing of dictation that comprised the original manuscript. We recognize critical assistance from Corrie Wickersham in retrieving an up-to-date accurate list of the Dingman Society members so we might contact them. We also received important typing and setup advice from Cindy Cooke. The preparation of the manuscript for this book would have been impossible without the guidance and support of Dr. Bob Parnes, our indispensable computer advisor. We are extremely grateful for the kindness, availability, and expertise of Chris Hedly, a fabulous graphic designer at Michigan MultiMedia. His skill and advice were invaluable in the management of all the photographs we were fortunate to get permission to use. We appreciate the encouragement and strong support of Nadine Lewis, the Plastic Surgery Section Administrator, during publishing negotiations. We are grateful for all the guidance and help in the final editing and publishing process from Allison Peters, Amanda Karby, and Jason Colman of Michigan Publishing Services. Bob Parnes, PhD provided essential computer expertise and invaluable assistance.

We are especially grateful for the excellent personal recollections from Drs. John Markley, Eric Austad, and Haskell Newman on subjects of great significance to our story from their respective areas of expertise. Dr. Paul Izenberg deserves special thanks, not only for his many personal recollections but also for his service in thoroughly editing the entire clinical section and giving us profound new insights in several categories that added greatly to the text. We also want to acknowledge Jeremiah (Jerry) Turcotte, MD, for providing access to the annual reports of the plastic surgery section from 1966 to 1975, which gave us accurate historical information.

We are very grateful to all those who contributed personal photographs to our project, including Bob Wilensky, Gary Nobel, Siggy Thorvaldsson, Ron Wexler, Richard Anderson, Harvey Weiss, David Dingman, Ann Chase, Terry Cromwell, Richard Sarns, Martha McClatchey, and Jim Norris. We hope to create an Ann Arbor Plastic Surgery Archive with all the photographs contributed for this project. We owe a debt of gratitude to Bob Gilman who contributed several copies of photographs that Joseph Murray had generously given to him from his collection at the Countway Library at Harvard Medical School. We wish to thank the Bentley Historical Library for their willingness to retrieve and for giving us permission to use three photographs from their collections. We also wish to thank Sister Yvonne Gellise, senior advisor for governance, for her permission to use three photographs from *The Healing Mission: The Practice of Medicine at SJMH 1911–1999*. We are also grateful to Cozy Grabb for providing us with copies of two photographs of Bill Grabb's balloon in action.

Finally, we are forever indebted to the many residents, fellows, and former faculty who took the time to contribute personal memories and anecdotes that have enlivened and enriched our history enormously.

CHAPTER ONE

# Early Influences on the Development of Plastic Surgery in Ann Arbor, Michigan

Our story begins at a time when two major influences were at work in the development of plastic surgery in Ann Arbor and in Michigan. One of the influences was the experience gained by exposure to the mutilating facial and extremity injuries suffered in World War I in Europe. "A European war, fought 5000 miles from home, triggered the development of plastic surgery in Michigan. For it was World War I, with its mass casualties having a high percentage of head and neck injuries, that created the need for more dynamic management of these problems. At first these patients would be treated abroad, particularly in England, but soon this knowledge and skill would span the Atlantic Ocean and come to the Great Lakes—especially to the state of Michigan."[1]

> Early in WWI it became evident to the Allies that a center should be developed where facial and other injuries involving large areas of tissue loss could be treated. Dr. Harold Gillies, a young enthusiastic otolaryngologist in the British Army, was designated to develop such a facility. Although Gillies had little experience in trauma surgery, he attacked the multiple problems with enthusiasm, courage and imagination. Reports of Gillies brilliant work reached North America and several American and Canadian physicians (such as Dr. Ferris Smith of Grand Rapids, MI [see Photo 1]), who were sympathetic with the British cause went to England, before America became involved in the conflict, to join Gillies' Maxillofacial unit.[2]

In 1916, Smith's father, Samuel, who was a US senator, arranged for Ferris to join Dr. Gillies in England. Dr. Smith became a captain in the Royal Medical Corps in England and practiced plastic surgery at the Queens Hospital, London. After the war, in 1918, Dr. Smith returned to Grand Rapids, Michigan, to start his plastic surgery practice.

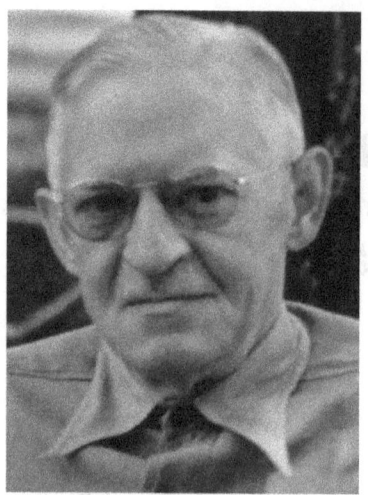

Photo 1: Dr. Ferris Smith.

The second influence happened when some oral surgeons, wanting to add to their surgical expertise and credentials, attended medical school and received their MD degree in addition to their existing DDS degrees. Among these was Dr. John Kemper. This allowed him to gain a wider experience in maxillofacial surgery. Dr. Reed O. Dingman, DDS, MD, also an oral surgeon, joined Dr. Kemper's practice in Ann Arbor. He then completed a formal plastic surgery preceptorship with Dr. Smith in Grand Rapids. Thus, he is an outstanding example of a pioneering plastic surgeon who was a product of both of these influences.

## John W. Kemper, MD (1891–1952)

In 1923, Dr. Kemper, an oral surgeon from Detroit, Michigan, enrolled in the University of Michigan (UM) Medical School and received his MD in 1927. During his second year of residency training in obstetrics and gynecology, he was invited by Dr. Chalmers J. Lyons, chair of the oral surgery department, to join the faculty at the UM Dental School as an instructor. As a result, in 1929, Dr. Kemper joined the dental faculty and discontinued his obstetric and gynecological training. Upon the death of Dr. Lyons in 1935, Dr. Kemper (Photo 2) was promoted to full professor and subsequently became head of the Department of Oral Surgery and a consultant at the University Hospital. He became very proficient in the management of patients with cleft lip and palate deformities as well as those with face and jaw lesions. In 1946, he presented a talk titled, "The Responsibility of the Surgeon in Treating Palatal and Related Defects."[3] He clearly outlined many of the basic responsibilities for

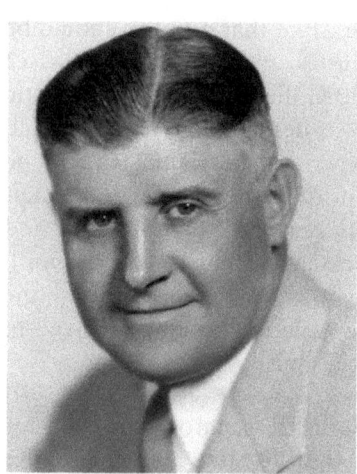

Photo 2: John W. Kemper (photo courtesy: Bentley Historical Library, University of Michigan).

surgeons in the care of cleft palate patients that were eventually taught to us by Dr. Dingman, twenty years after this presentation. It highlights the sophisticated knowledge, experience, and humanity that Dr. Kemper demonstrated in 1946.

In 1937, Dr. Kemper became a founding member of the American Board of Plastic Surgery and a member of the American Association of Plastic Surgery, which was the first plastic surgery society in the United States. He was also very influential in the American Society of Maxillofacial Surgeons and was elected as its second president in 1948. His excellent work paved the way for plastic surgery to enter into the medical school curriculum and eventually led to a Section of Plastic Surgery within the UM Department of Surgery. Dr. Kemper served as the chairman for the Department of Oral Surgery until his sudden death in 1952. "John Kemper was a large man with a great heart, a friendly smile, a person of sincerity with a fine sense of fairness. His wise counsel was sought by his associates and his students. He was a big, handsome, friendly person loved by his students, colleagues and patients."[4]

## Reed O. Dingman, MD, DDS (1906–85)

Dr. Reed O. Dingman grew up in Detroit, Michigan (Photo 3). He went to Southwestern High School and then graduated from Wayne State University. He received his AB degree from the UM in 1928 and his DDS degree from the UM Dental School in 1931. In 1932, he completed a master's degree in oral surgery and became an assistant professor in the Department of Oral Surgery. In addition, in 1932, he enrolled in the UM Medical School, receiving his MD degree in 1936. From 1936 to 1937, Dr. Dingman completed a straight surgery internship at Barnes Hospital in St. Louis, Missouri, under Dr. Minot Fryer. After his internship, he was a resident in oral and maxillofacial surgery at the Geisinger Memorial Clinic in Danville, Pennsylvania, from 1937 to 1939. In 1940, he returned to Ann Arbor, accepted a position as assistant professor in the UM Dental School, and became an assistant to Dr. John Kemper. He also served as a preceptor in plastic surgery at the medical school.

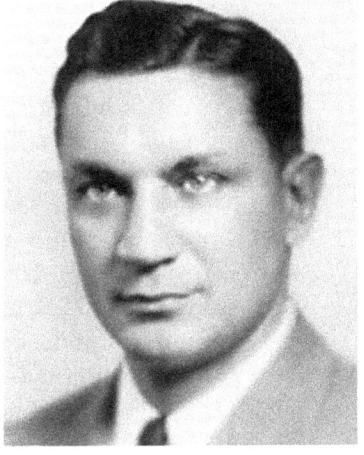

Photo 3: Reed O. Dingman, DDS, MD (c. late 1930s).

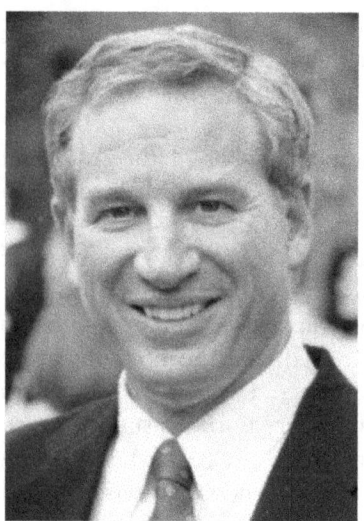

Photo 4: David Dingman.

In 1945, as he felt a need for more formal training, he enrolled as a resident in plastic surgery for one year under Dr. Ferris Smith at Blodgett Hospital in Grand Rapids, Michigan. David (Photo 4), Dr. Dingman's son, related to me his recollection that it was during his father's time in Grand Rapids in training with Dr. Smith that the accident occurred in which Dr. Smith was hit by a car and subsequently suffered very severe and disabling injuries. According to Dave, his father had to take over a lot of Dr. Smith's practice in Grand Rapids even while he was still completing his training.[5] In 1946, Dr. Dingman returned to Ann Arbor, continuing as associate professor of oral surgery, and joined Dr. Kemper in a private plastic surgery practice at Saint Joseph Mercy Hospital (SJMH) in Ann Arbor (see Photo 5).

They both felt that there was a need for a formal plastic surgical training experience in Ann Arbor. In his own words, Dr. Dingman explained the origins of the original preceptorship at SJMH:

> Following the end of the Second World War, many young men were seeking places in which to train and get experience in plastic and reconstructive surgery. Although there was no formal training program at the University of Michigan, Dr. Kemper and I in 1948 developed a preceptee program for a one- or two-year period to accommodate some of those who wished to come to Ann Arbor. Appointments were to SJMH in Ann Arbor, where we had private patients. Preceptees also worked in the Department of Oral Surgery at University Hospital. Dr. Joseph Ewing of Akron, Ohio, was one of the first to come to Ann Arbor on this basis. He remained for a year and was followed by Drs. Howard Billman, Clyde Litton (1948), Wilmer Hansen (1952), and Paul Natvig (1955). Although this was not an approved residency training program at the time, our trainees were given recognition as preceptees and permitted to sit for examination by the American Board of Plastic Surgery.[6]

Circumstances following Dr. Kemper's sudden death in 1952 had a profound influence on the history of plastic surgery and its relationship with

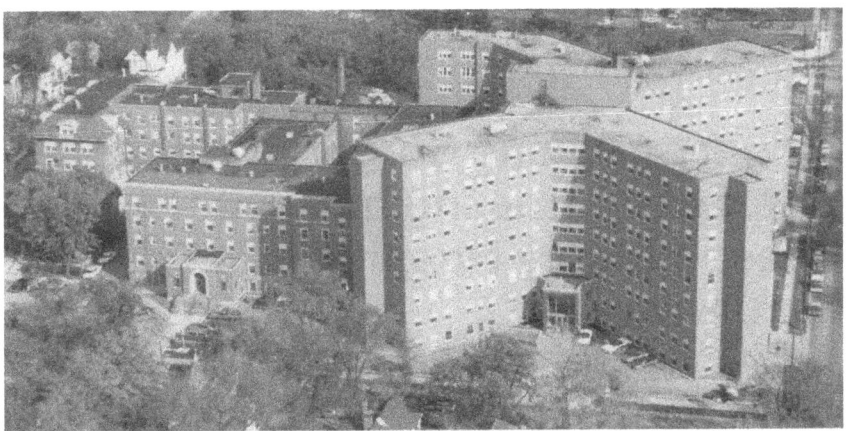

Photo 5: Saint Joseph Mercy Hospital (c. 1955).

the UM Dental School. Dr. Dingman was invited to succeed Dr. Kemper as the chairman of the Department of Oral Surgery at the dental school, but he declined this offer and instead accepted a position as an assistant professor in the Department of Surgery at the Medical Center. This decision was thought to be the cause of some resentment over the years within the dental school, specifically within the oral surgery department. It seems Dr. Dingman had a vision that the best chance of ultimately forming a plastic surgery section had to come from within the Department of Surgery at the university by providing good patient care as well as education. He felt that Dr. Frederick Coller, chairman of the Department of Surgery (Photo 6), wanted plastic surgery exposure in the surgery department to enhance teaching for the general surgery residents.

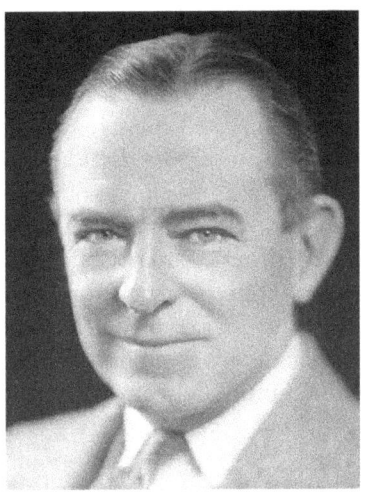

Photo 6: Frederick A. Coller, MD.

CHAPTER TWO

# Origin of Plastic Surgery Residency Training at Saint Joseph Mercy Hospital in Ann Arbor

From 1955 to 1957, while Dr. Paul Natvig was serving his preceptee time, he became a prime mover along with Dr. Dingman in an effort to establish an approved residency at Saint Joseph Mercy Hospital (SJMH) that could be affiliated with the surgery department at the UM. Sister Mary Xavier Shields (Photo 7), the head administrator at SJMH, had become enthusiastic about plastic surgery after Dr. Dingman removed an "unsightly" hemangioma from her own sister's lip. She became aware of many other dramatic plastic surgery cases. Her help and guidance were essential in the formation of the new residency program. Progress toward this objective evolved, and after the necessary data were compiled, an application was submitted to the Joint Commission on Residency Training, which ultimately gave approval in 1957 for a two-year residency for one trainee a year. Dr. Natvig (Photo 8) received the first certificate when he

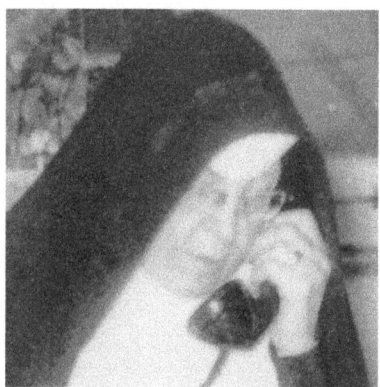

Photo 7: Sister Mary Xavier Shields.

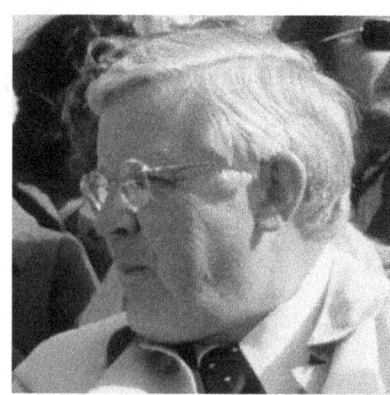

Photo 8: Paul Natvig, MD.

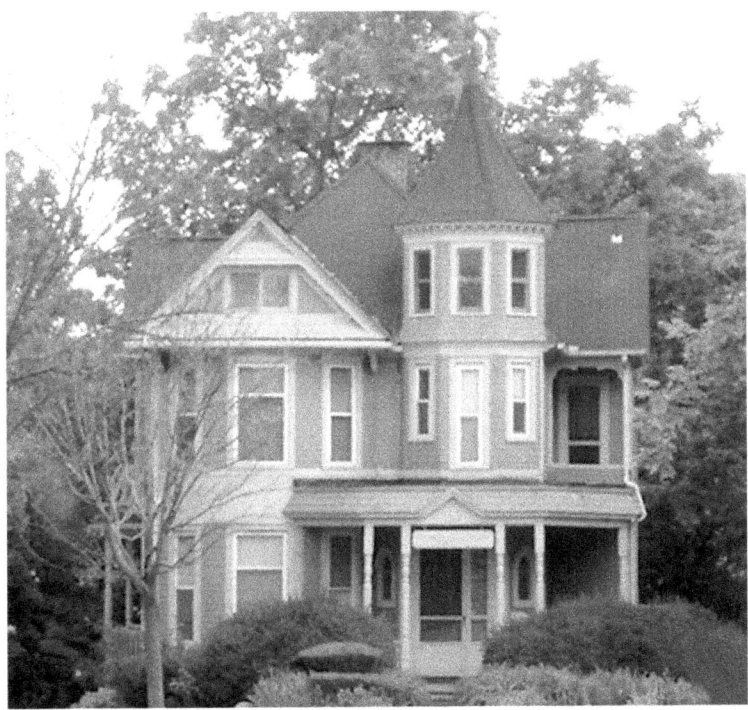

*Photo 9:* House behind SJMH resembling the one housing the surgical laboratory at SJMH.

completed his training, which was signed by both Dr. Frederick A. Coller and Sister Mary Xavier. The latter continued to be a strong supporter of the new program and made sure that it received adequate financial support, designated beds, and adequate operating room (OR) time, as well as laboratory space in an adjoining building on site (see Photo 9). Dr. John Tipton and Dr. Dingman published a report on their research project concerning the effects of wound healing in germ-free animals in 1966.[1] John had been a general surgery resident at SJMH, prior to starting his plastic surgery residency there in 1963. This project is a good example of the support that Sister Xavier extended to research at the residency program at SJMH. It was a complex project requiring a lot of specialized housing to keep the animals germ free from birth.

From 1958 to 1964, six residents were trained, including Dr. William C. Grabb (Photo 10). Bill grew up in Fairport, New York, where he attended high school. He then attended Michigan State University, followed by an internship at Ohio State. Then he became a lifetime "Michigan Man" when he began his three-year surgery residency at the University of Michigan (UM) interrupted by two years in the US Air Force Medical Corps. In 1954, early in his general surgery residency at the university, Grabb had

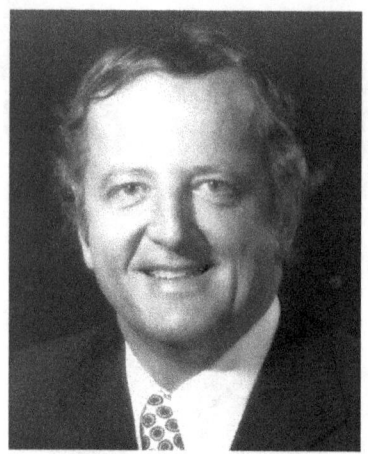

Photo 10: William C. Grabb, MD.

approached Dr. Dingman, and the event is best conveyed in Dr. Dingman's own words from his eulogy for Dr. Grabb after his sudden death in 1982:

In the fall of 1954, as I was walking in the hallway at university hospital, I was approached by a handsome young resident with an engaging smile who asked politely if he could have a few words with me. In our brief conversation that followed he informed me that he would like to become a plastic surgeon and have his training on my service, which at that time, was based at St. Joseph Mercy Hospital but was affiliated with university hospital. In response to my question of why he wanted to become a plastic surgeon, Bill Grabb gave me several good reasons: he wished to be a surgeon; he liked the challenges of reconstructive surgery; he felt that many problems in plastic surgery had not yet been solved; there was a great opportunity for creative thinking and research; and he hoped eventually to become a teacher. These were all excellent reasons and indicated motivation to me that appeared most promising. He was invited to my office to discuss this in greater detail; and during the next three years while he was a resident in general surgery at University Hospital, we had several discussions about his continuing interest in plastic surgery. Finally Bill was selected from among other applicants to begin training with me.[2]

Dr. Grabb completed the residency program in 1961 and stayed on as Dr. Dingman's partner and as a clinical instructor in the Department of Surgery at Michigan. There continued to be one new resident a year in the two-year program. Several additional fellows spent just one year in the program. The program flourished in close liaison with the University of Michigan Department of Surgery, and many general surgery trainees rotated on plastic surgery at SJMH for one to two months.

## Introduction of Robert M. Oneal to Plastic Surgery

I grew up on the north shore of Chicago and knew I wanted to be a physician at nine years of age. I attended three years of undergraduate/premed at Dartmouth and then the first two years of medical school. My last two years were at Harvard. I then came to UM Hospital in Ann Arbor for a

> # The Principles and Art of
> # PLASTIC SURGERY
>
> *By*
> ### SIR HAROLD GILLIES, C.B.E., F.R.C.S.
> *and*
> ### D. RALPH MILLARD, JR., M.D.
> Fellow of the American College of Surgeons. Diplomate, American Board of Plastic Surgery. Associate Clinical Professor, University of Miami School of Medicine
>
> *Chapter on Anaesthesia by* IVAN MAGILL, C.V.O., F.F.A.R.C.S.
>
> *With a Foreword by* JEROME PIERCE WEBSTER, M.D.
> Professor of Clinical Surgery, College of Physicians and Surgeons, Columbia University

Photo 11: Title page of *The Principles and Art of Plastic Surgery*.

mixed surgery internship followed by a general surgery residency. (On a personal note, my father-in-law trained in thoracic surgery at UM in the 1930s, and he and my wife's mother thought Ann Arbor would be a fine place to live and raise a family.) It was during my third year of general surgery residency at the UM Hospital, in 1962, that I had the opportunity to meet Dr. Dingman for the first time while caring for his patients. Dr. Dingman admitted both "charity" adults and children to the university hospital, and they were cared for by the residents on the general surgery service. During this time, I became intrigued with plastic surgery in a way that changed the course of my professional life forever. Dr. Dingman introduced me to a book, *The Principles and Art of Plastic Surgery*, by Sir Harold Gillies and Dr. Ralph Millard Jr. (see Photo 11).[3]

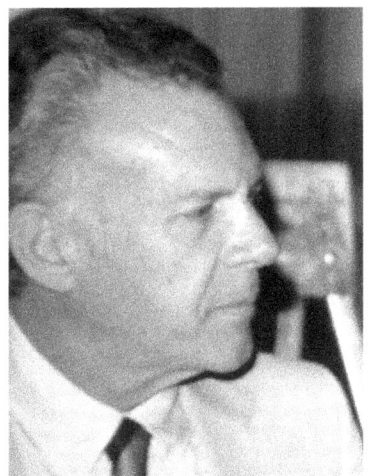

Photo 12: D. Ralph Millard, MD.

Dr. Millard (Photo 12), following his training, worked in England with Dr. Gillies, who had extensive experience in providing plastic surgery to war-injured patients. Dr. Millard helped Dr. Gillies collect all his work and ideas into a two-volume textbook that became an early "bible" of plastic surgery. The book was a great inspiration to me and one of the factors, in addition to the experience of working with Dr. Dingman in the OR, that ultimately influenced me in shifting from a career in general surgery to one in plastic surgery. Dr. Dingman had offered some political support to Dr. Millard during his early years in practice, and they remained close friends throughout their careers. It was a thrill for me to meet Dr. Millard when he was invited to Michigan as one of the first visiting professors in the new plastic surgery section in 1966. Another inspiration was the friendship I developed with Bill Grabb during my final years in general surgery residency. He inspired my interest in hand surgery and gave me copies of many slides of various hand injuries that I might use for teaching at the University of Nebraska when I joined the faculty there in 1963. My admiration for Bill was one of the factors responsible for my return to Ann Arbor.

CHAPTER THREE

# Creation of the Section of Plastic Surgery in the University of Michigan Department of Surgery

The narrative continues with the background story of the formation of the University of Michigan (UM) plastic surgery section finalized in 1964. Then follows discussion of the growth of the section up to Dr. Dingman's (ROD) retirement as section head in 1975 and Dr. Grabb's (WCG) succession.

Although there was a plastic surgery residency at Saint Joseph Mercy Hospital (SJMH) affiliated with the Department of Surgery at the UM, there remained a long road ahead to finalizing a Section of Plastic Surgery within the surgery department at the UM Hospital (see Photo 13).

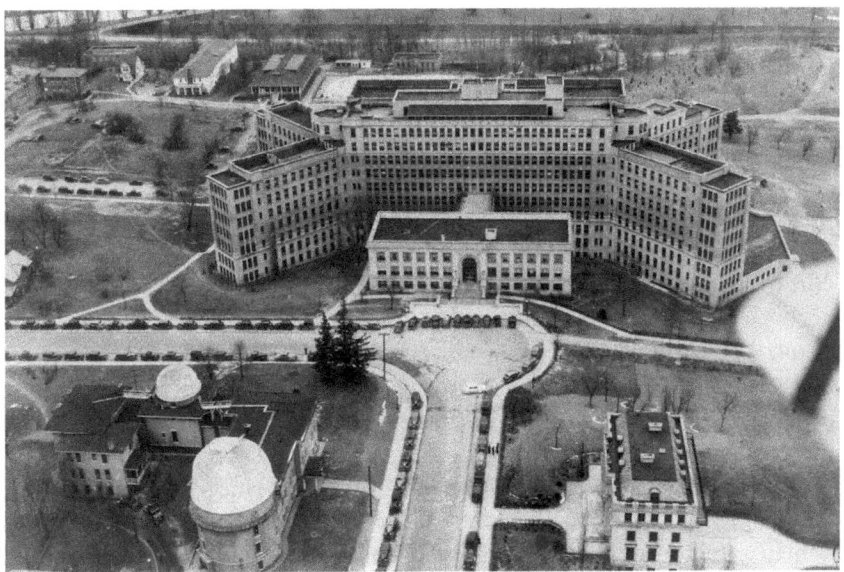

*Photo 13:* University of Michigan Hospital: historic Detroit Observatory on the left and the Simpson Memorial Building on the right. (Photo courtesy of the Bentley Historical Library, University of Michigan.)

11

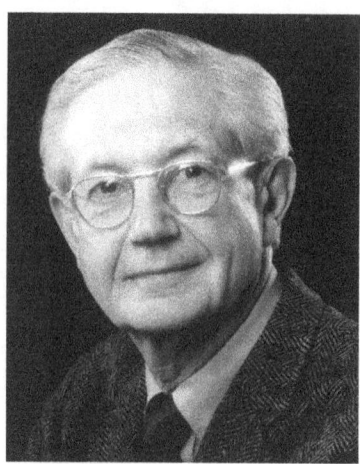

Photo 14: Charles Gardner Child III, MD, chairman of the Department of Surgery (1959–1974).

There was resistance to its formation because some in the surgery department felt that the most significant plastic surgery procedures could be done by well-trained general surgeons. There was also resistance from the otolaryngology (ENT) department and the oral surgery section within the Department of Surgery.

In 1959, Dr. Charles Gardner Child III (Photo 14) became chairman of the Department of Surgery following the retirement of Dr. Coller in 1958. This created an opportunity for Dr. Dingman to pursue the idea of a Section of Plastic Surgery within the UM Department of Surgery. As far as the American Board of Plastic Surgery was concerned, the residency was already established through the program at SJMH and it was the university issue that had to be finalized. Owing to Dr. Child's previous administrative experience at both Cornell and Tufts Medical Schools, prior to coming to the UM, he had gained appreciation for important contributions to teaching, research, and patient care that a well-organized Section of Plastic Surgery could provide. He facilitated discussion between Dr. Dingman andCed Dr. Walter Work, chairman of otolaryngology, and Dr. James Hayward, chairman of oral surgery, all of whom had strong personalities. The relationship with oral surgery was particularly complicated because of some residual resentment over Dr. Dingman's previous decision back in 1952 to reject the offer of chairmanship of oral surgery. It took an extended period of meetings, conferences, and faculty votes during the years from 1960 to 1964 to achieve the compromises necessary to allow formation of the Section of Plastic Surgery in early 1964. Dr. Dingman was then appointed associate professor of surgery and section head of plastic surgery. The existing residency training program at SJMH was fully integrated into the section and remains an integral partner in the UM plastic surgery training program to this day.

The "grand compromise" among the plastic surgery, oral surgery, and ENT that was worked out under the guidance of Dr. Child was a major factor in plastic surgery becoming an official section within the Department of Surgery. The agreement contained the following compromises: plastic surgery was to assume the care of all infants with primary cleft lip deformities admitted to the UM Hospital; palate repairs were to be divided evenly between plastic and oral surgery; plastic surgery and ENT would alternate call in the emergency room for facial soft tissue trauma and fractures; and oral surgery was to be called for isolated mandibular fractures and to share in the care of patients with multiple fractures when the mandible was involved. Recalling Dr. Child's wise mediation over this originally seeming insolvable conflict makes one realize how important it is to strive for compromises that can result in a win-win solution. What was achieved was a grand outcome: *The Section of Plastic Surgery at the UM*.

## Early History of the New Section of Plastic Surgery at the UM

Dr. Grabb continued as an assistant professor at the university after the section was formed and also maintained his private practice at SJMH. He was a very active and productive faculty member along with Dr. Dingman in the training of the residents. The residency program within the newly formed section was originally approved for two trainees per year. Dr. John Tipton (Photo 15) had started the residency at SJMH in 1963. In 1964, he was to become the second-year resident at UM. Late in 1963, Dr. Dingman had called me at 6:00 a.m. in Omaha, where I had taken a teaching position in general surgery at the University of Nebraska having completed my general surgery residency. He told me that he had another opening for the residency program now that the section had been formed and offered me a position (Photo 16). I accepted and joined Dr. Don Davis (Photo 17), who had been appointed to the preexisting SJMH program, as a first year co-resident. In 1966, Dr. Dingman expanded the program to three trainees per year. Frequently, there was a Ford Hospital plastic surgery resident for a six-month rotation and an international fellow for six to twelve months.

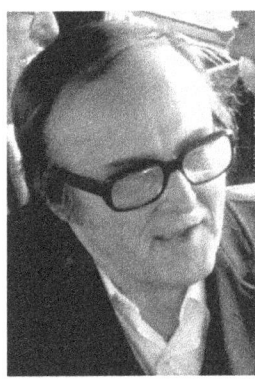

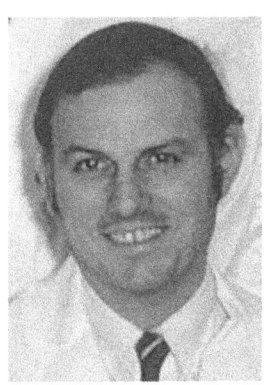

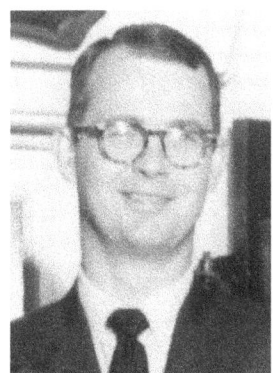

Photo 15:
John B. Tipton, MD.

Photo 16:
Robert M. Oneal, MD.

Photo 17:
Don G. Davis, MD.

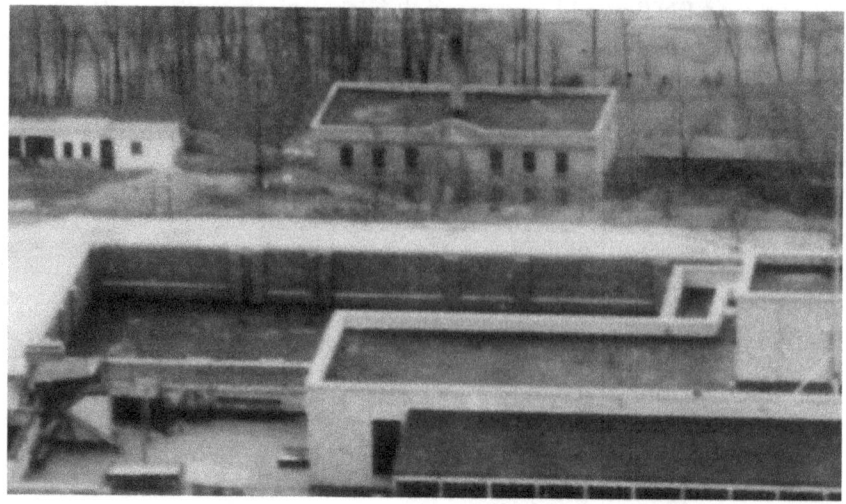

*Photo 18:* North Outpatient Building (NOB) directly north of the main hospital.

The first offices and clinic of the university program, after the section was officially formed, were located in the North Outpatient Building (NOB; see Photo 18). This was a small building directly north of the main hospital, and it was originally a readjustment center for returning World War II veterans. We have a copy of the list of "essentials" that Dr. Dingman made for establishing the new office: a key, a name on the door, paint on the walls, a Dictaphone, and a rack for forms. These minimal requirements were a big step-up from his previous office at the university, which had consisted of a coat rack with a shelf on top to store charts and books. There were two main office rooms, both of which had previously been bedrooms. One was Dr. Dingman's office and the other a resident/faculty office for six residents, two faculty members, and a nurse. There was a secretarial office in between.

Lauralee Lutz became the section head secretary in 1968 and loyally continued in the position for twenty years. She acquired the affectionate nickname, "L3" (Photo 19). There were also two patient-examining rooms across the hall with a part-time registered nurse who helped with patients during office hours. Dr. Dingman was a stickler

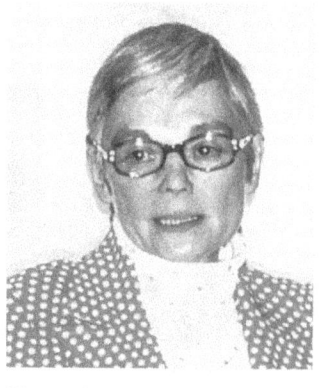

*Photo 19:* Lauralee Lutz.

about personal appearance. One of his famous admonitions was, "If you are a professional, look and act like one." His recommendations to achieve that included the following: no facial hair, press your pants, get periodic haircuts, clean white coat at all times, wear a shirt and tie, and no Hawaiian sport shirts (ever). The "no facial hair" was gradually modified as social norms changed but he continued to demand shined shoes. One of L3's most vivid memories of our time in the NOB was seeing the mandatory shoe shine box being shared by both residents and faculty polishing their shoes.[1]

Dr. Wexler's (resident, 1970–72) recollections of L3:

> Our lovely secretary Lauralee Lutz was the pivot and the anchor of the section life. She took care of everything needed and I knew, as the rest of us residents did, that we could bring to L-3 any question or problem and she would come with the appropriate solution—after discussing it "with the authorities" . . . Once I mentioned to her that a recommendation letter ROD wrote for me was beautifully written, and L-3 said: "Well, actually I wrote it!" . . . "How come?" I asked. "Well," she said, "it is rather easy, I, sit backward, pretending I am ROD himself dictating the letter and the letter is being printed by itself! Simple, you see???!!!" Of course, ROD made slight corrections and added his impressive signature. L-3 brought much kindness and gentleness to her office with her love to everything and everybody around her with the beloved amaryllis on her desk, and the globe map in which every former resident and fellow was marked with a little flag.[2]

The plastic surgery section, on the first floor of NOB, was one of three other clinical services and offices in this revamped building. A well-baby clinic was next to us on the first floor, and around the corner near the library were emeritus professors' offices for Dr. Bruce Fralich, longtime head of ophthalmology, and Dr. Henry Ransom, who had been acting head of the surgery department. On the second floor were the allergy department and several psychology and psychiatry offices.

The basement housed the Department of Medical Illustration, headed by Gerald Hodge (Photo 20). Denis Lee and several other talented artists were also members of

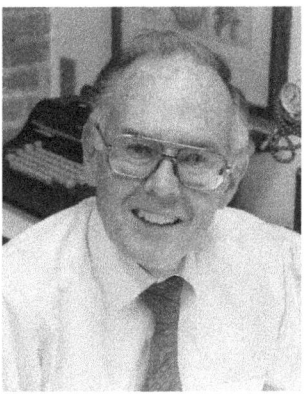

Photo 20: Gerald P. Hodge. (Photo courtesy of the Bentley Historical Library, University of Michigan.)

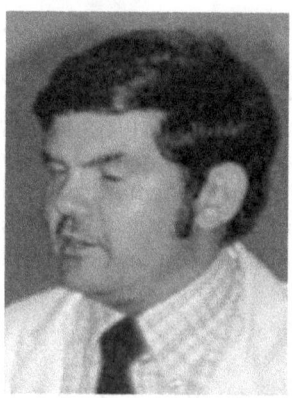

Photo 21: Denis Lee.

that department. We had a close liaison with them on many of the papers and books that plastic surgery was involved in. Often, one of them would join us in the operating room (OR) to gain a more accurate vision of the anatomic structure or surgical manipulation they would be depicting. Over the years, a strong sense of mutual respect had developed between the two services. Dr. Dingman had always appreciated artwork and the artistic spirit. The origins of the medical sculpture program are documented from annual section reports 70–71 and 72–73 written by Dr. Dingman:

In early spring, 1971, a Medical Sculpture Service was begun in cooperation with Mr. Denis Lee [Photo 21] and Professor Gerard P. Hodge of the Department of Medical and Biological Illustration. This new service offers prosthetic correction for facial disfigurement, particularly in patients who are not considered as operative candidates because of age or extent of their facial deformity. Patient referrals are expected from all departments and sections of the Medical Center as well as from outside physicians. Already Mr. Lee, who had received special training in constructing medical prostheses, has created prostheses for patients lacking a nose, ear, part of a cheek, partial skull defect, and one patient with pectus excavatum. In five months, Mr. Lee had seen twenty-four patients. By 1973, Mr. Lee had treated patients from all the UM affiliated hospitals and from others in the Midwest area. During this fiscal year Mr. Lee constructed 34 prostheses.[3]

The program continued successfully within the plastic surgery section for many years and was appreciated by many grateful patients.

In 1976, the plastic surgery offices moved to the seventh floor of the main outpatient building, which is now the Med Inn (see Photo 22). The offices occupied an entire corridor. Plastic surgery shared the floor with general surgery, thoracic surgery, and the Department of Surgery offices. In this new location, there was a large waiting room that was decorated much like a living room—a way to help make patients feel more comfortable. There were several exam rooms, faculty offices, a minor surgery room, a nurse's office, and, eventually, an exam room containing a laser to treat hemangiomas. The Reed O. Dingman Library (an acknowledgment of Dr. Dingman's commitment to the heritage of plastic surgery) occupied its own room and contained a wide selection of the important plastic

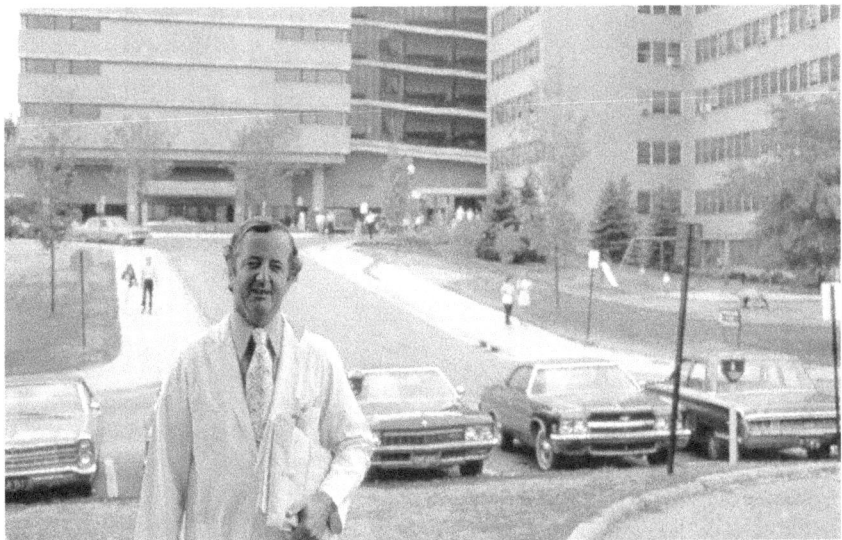

*Photo 22:* Bill Grabb, with manuscript in hand, facing NOB; new Mott Children's Hospital directly behind him and the Outpatient Building to his left.

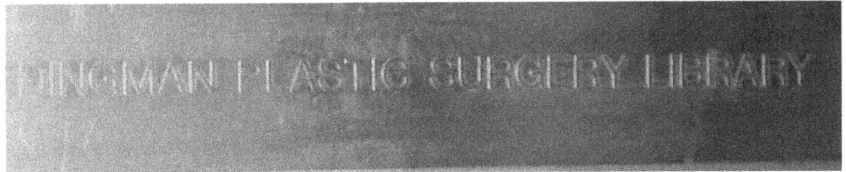

*Photo 23:* Plaque for Reed O. Dingman Library.

surgery texts, journals, and a panel of famous quotations (see Photos 23 and 24). It was popular and used frequently by faculty, residents, and students. The contents of the library have since been moved and combined with the Department of Surgery library in the Taubman Building.

Lauralee Lutz, our long-standing secretary of the section, continued to be the "power behind the throne" to both Drs. Dingman and Grabb. She now had some secretarial help as the clinic size had grown and operating schedule expanded. There was great camaraderie among the faculty, secretaries, and

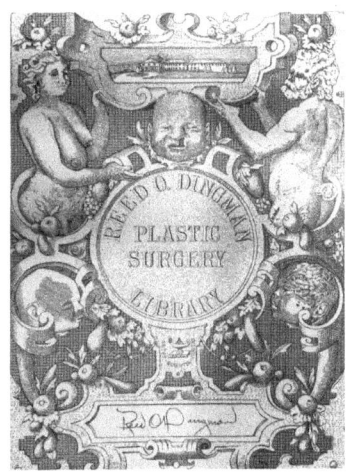

*Photo 24:* Bookmark for Reed O. Dingman Library.

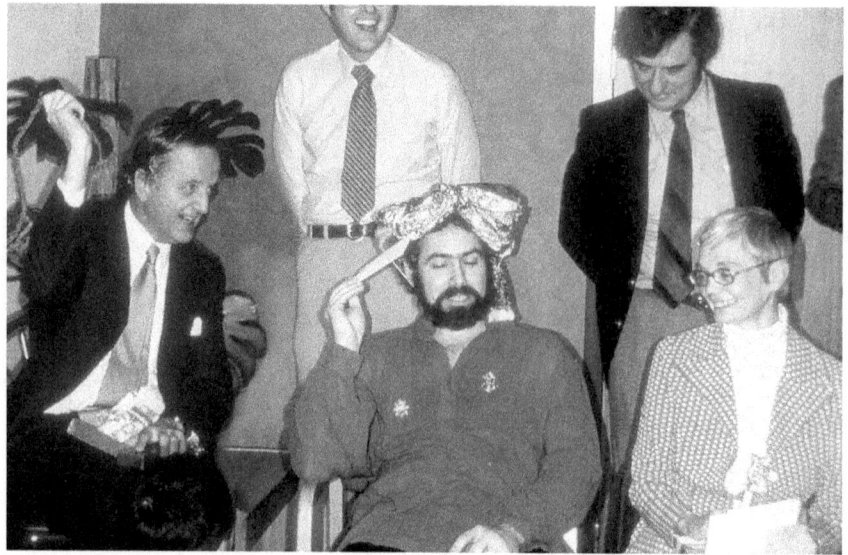

*Photo 25:* Holiday party with Dr. Grabb animated and Dr. Paul Izenberg impersonating Karmak the Great.

residents, and we always had a holiday party. The holiday parties were held in the section offices until a student guest had a little too much wine and we had to move the party locations to private homes (see Photo 25).

### Additional Faculty Appointments to the New Section

Dr. John B. Tipton: In 1965, John opened a practice in Ann Arbor, and his primary teaching activities were at SJMH where he had his private patients. He was an excellent surgeon, very well read, and an original thinker. He was an important part of the teaching programs both in the OR and in conferences. He decided to start a practice in Palm Springs, California, partly for health reasons, and left Ann Arbor in 1969.

Dr. Robert M. Oneal (RMO): When I completed my residency in 1966, Dr. Dingman appointed me as instructor in the Section of Plastic Surgery. I also saw private patients together with Drs. Grabb and Dingman at the 221 N. Ingalls Street office across the street from old SJMH. After three years, I was promoted to clinical associate professor. I eventually started my own practice, with Dr. Dingman's blessing, in downtown Ann Arbor with an office on the twenty-fifth floor of the Tower Plaza in 1969 and continued my part-time teaching responsibilities.

Ron Wexler (resident, 1970–72) recollected the three faculty members at the time of his training:

> I admire the outstanding collaboration among our three staff members, ROD, WCG, and RMO—the King, the Crown Prince and the Prince. I know that the "Section of Plastic Surgery" was not a monarchy, it was a voluntary hierarchy, in which mutual respect, discipline, professionalism, and knowledge were the binding glue. ROD, the King. He was a "doer." He loved operating and I loved working with him. He was open-minded and listened to any remark or suggestion, even from a first-year resident. He was a hard worker. He could work endlessly. When we were at his office, seeing all his patients, embedded in soft evening music, he would eat an olive between cases and around 11 p.m. he would say: "OK boys, you can have the rest of the day off," provided we were not on call for the emergency room.
> 
> WCG was the scholar surgeon. When any of the residents would come up with an idea, he would ask, "Did you check all the literature to see if it had been previously mentioned?" He emphasized, nonstop, the need to be knowledgeable . . . He loved all the fascinating advances in plastic surgery and was thrilled to share it with us. (We all became familiar with WCG's "Ten Most Wanted" list of the classics or recent literature, and then a couple of months later, he would come out with the second list to keep us on our toes [see A-8 in the appendix for these lists].)

Ron Wexler continued,

> RMO was an elegant surgeon. As he was just a bit older than us all, we looked at him as a friend and brother. He was very prudent and meticulous in his surgery and I remember once his rhinoplasty took a bit longer than expected. He looked at me and said, "Ron, remember, in one year nobody will ask you how long did the operation take, but everybody will ask you how the result is!" I used this saying hundreds of times since, in my teaching [see Photos 26 and 27].[4]

Dr. John M. Markley Jr. joined the UM faculty and my practice in 1974. I had known John both as a medical student and as a beginning surgical resident and had followed his career as a combined plastic surgery resident at Stanford under Dr. Robert Chase and then during a hand fellowship under Dr. William Littler in New York City. Dr. Dingman encouraged

20  *Creation of the Section of Plastic Surgery*

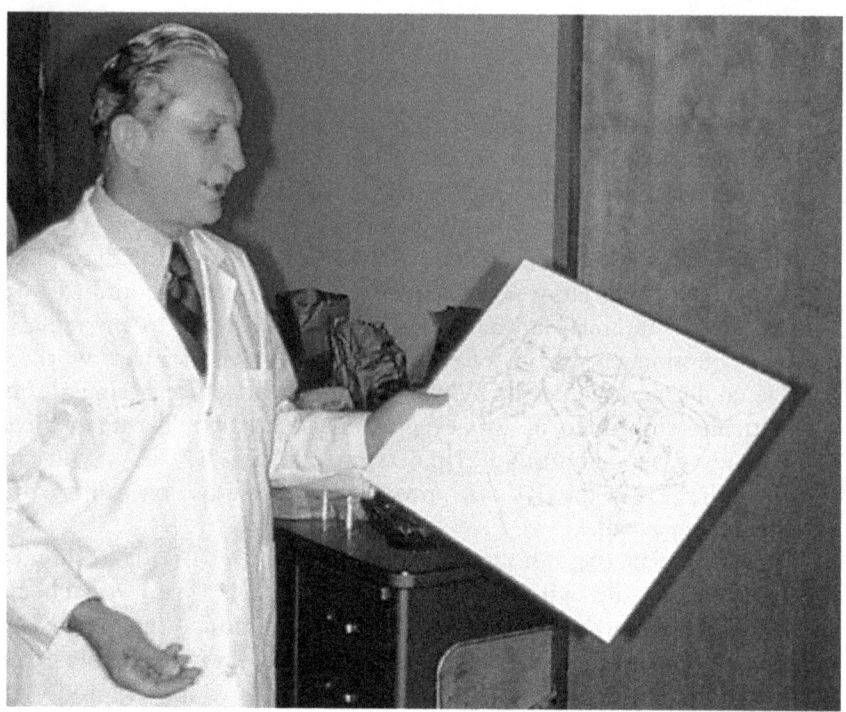

*Photo 26:* Dr. Dingman holding the "cartoon" drawn by Denis Lee of the faculty and L3.

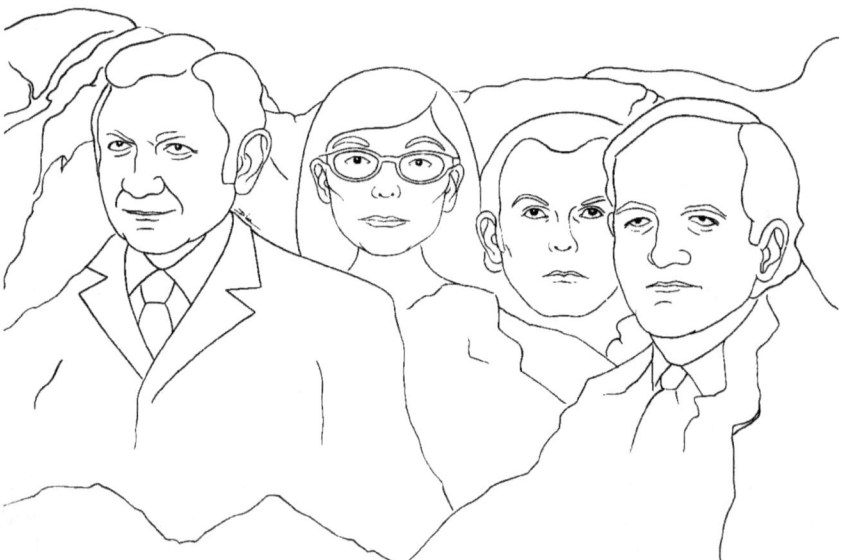

*Photo 27:* "Mt. Rushmore cartoon": Dr. Dingman, Lauralee Lutz, and Drs. Oneal and Grabb (from left to right).

John's return to Ann Arbor as he felt additional faculty was needed due to rapid growth of the section. I was thrilled that he wanted to come back to Ann Arbor, and so we teamed up as partners in our office in the Tower Plaza. Dr. Markley immediately became an important member of our faculty (Photo 28). His surgical skills and expertise in hand and microsurgery made him an essential addition to the program. He was also obviously a self-starter, as in John's own words, "During my Stanford residency in 1970, [during] a 6 month lab rotation, I taught myself microvascular technique in the empty but still equipped micro lab Harry Buncke left behind when he left Stanford. I visited him a couple times at his lab in Mountain View, and used some written material he had generated, and just taught myself, doing rat kidney transplants, end-end arterial, venous, and ureteral anastomoses. This led to doing a rat renal transplant immunologic study with the transplant surgeon at Stanford (Lucas) which was published in 1970."[5]

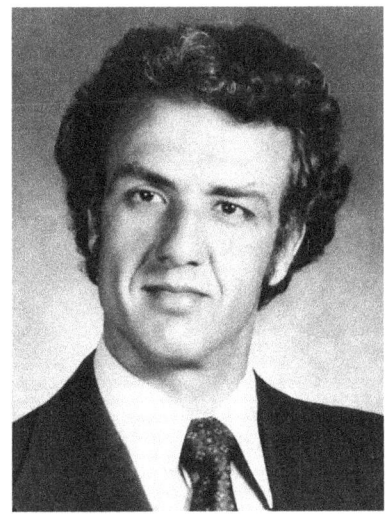

Photo 28: John M. Markley, MD.

## Two Interesting Aspects Unique to Early Years of the Residency Program

### 1. The Michigan-Maryland Connection

Dr. Robert Buxton had been a professor of general surgery at the UM and was recruited to become the chief of surgery at the University of Maryland. He had been one of the most popular faculty members, and everyone spoke highly of him at Michigan. The medical students at the time also knew him, and he, therefore, attracted several of them to Maryland for general surgery residency, including Dr. David Dingman (Dr. Dingman's son) and Dr. Ted Dodenhoff. This was crucial to Ted's future as he recalled:

> I first met Dr. Dingman through his son Dave, my close friend in Medical school. I knew him as more of a second father figure in my life at a time when I had no clue what kind of a career I was going to have after medical school. Once Dave and I reunited in General surgery at the University of Maryland, we began to realize that the

future of General Surgery was going to be bleak and Plastic Surgery offered a better future. Luckily, the program at Michigan was one of the best and the only place I had any chance to get into because of the late decision to seek a residency. I'm sure I got in mainly because Dr. Dingman knew me and felt confident that I would work out well in the program.[6]

From 1969 through 1975, we accepted into the program seven residents who, while training in general surgery at the University of Maryland, came to be interested in plastic surgery training at the UM. They were all very good surgeons and a great addition to the program. While Ted Dodenhoff was one of the residents, the others were Lenny Glass, Tom Hudak, Carl Berner, Grant Fairbanks, Gary Nobel, and Bob Wilensky.

## 2. Changes in the Board Requirements for Plastic Surgery Training

In 1971, the American Board of Plastic Surgery altered its requirement for residency training to include those who had become board-qualified in a surgical specialty other than general surgery. Dr. Dingman was very open and outspoken about accepting the best candidates who he thought could become excellent plastic surgeons. Because of his willingness to offer residency positions in the plastic surgery program to otolaryngologists who had completed their training, Dr. Dingman engendered a lot of criticism from some of his longtime plastic surgery friends.

Dr. John O'Connor (1972–74), who had his boards in otolaryngology and dentistry, was the first of these residents from other surgical specialties to enter the UM plastic surgery residency program. Others who entered the program between 1973 and 1986 included Drs. Dick Lawrence, Haskell Newman, Merle Olesen, Jack Gunter, Mike Watanabe, Erlan Duus, Richard Anderson, and Dick Pollock (all otolaryngology), while Drs. Robert Gilman (otolaryngology and dentistry), Bruce Novark (oral surgery), and Biff McCollum (orthopedics) rounded out the group. These highly trained specialty surgeons provided a unique experience for our faculty and the other residents who had not had this additional training. We valued their expertise in all aspects of dentistry and head and neck surgery, especially in rhinoplasty, facial fractures, and head and neck cancer treatment, as well as Dr. McCollum's expertise in the management of hand and wrist fractures.

CHAPTER FOUR

# Transitions in the Section of Plastic Surgery

The second decade of the Section of Plastic Surgery included some dramatic events: Reed O. Dingman's retirement, Bill Grabb replacing him, several new faculty appointments, Dr. Grabb's sudden and unexpected death in 1982, Dr. Dingman's return as acting head, a search for a new section head, and Dr. Dingman's death in December 1985, which closes the time frame of the narrative of this book.

## Dr. Dingman's Retirement as Section Head

In 1975, Dr. Dingman began his year-long "so-called" retirement furlough. He had been a very strong and highly respected leader since 1964. During his career, he was given many honors and was elected to many leadership positions, including president of the Society of Maxillofacial Surgeons; president of the Society of Plastic and Reconstructive Surgeons, as well as president of its Educational Foundation; and chairman of the American Board of Plastic Surgery. He was also honored by being selected as visiting professor in seventeen universities in the United States and around the world (Photo 29). It is both quite interesting and poignant to read Dr. Dingman's thoughts from the 1973–74 annual report to Dean John A. Gronvall, MD, which cataloged the section's progress during his tenure as section head:

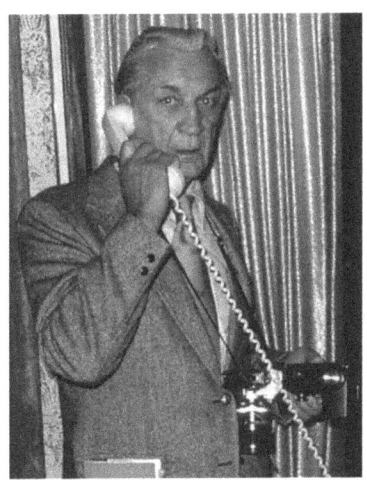

*Photo 29:* Dr. Dingman in his sixth-floor office in the outpatient building at the university hospital, on the phone holding a camera.

23

This report concludes the tenth year since the establishment of the Section of Plastic Surgery at the University of Michigan. During this period, the Section of Plastic Surgery has become a well-integrated and important part of the teaching of surgery in the Medical School. The section is well known throughout the State of Michigan as a center for the provision of plastic surgery care, research, and teaching. It has been unofficially regarded as being an outstanding resident training program in plastic surgery. We have been able to maintain high standards as prerequisites for training in our program and have attracted outstanding candidates from all parts of the world.[1]

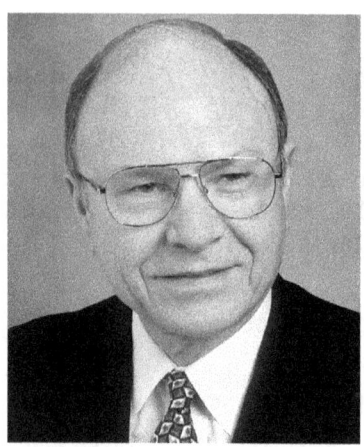

Photo 30: Jeremiah Turcotte, MD.

Dr. Dingman's thoughts on his successor and his upcoming retirement are included in the 1974–75 annual report of the section to Department Chairman Jeremiah G. Turcotte, MD, a widely respected transplant surgeon and a good friend of all of us in plastic surgery (Photo 30). Dr. Dingman wrote, "A Search Committee appointed by Dr. Turcotte, after a nationwide search for Dr. Dingman's successor, recommended Dr. William C. Grabb as the most qualified surgeon to assume the position of new Head of the Section of Plastic Surgery. Negotiations with the Department of Surgery and the Medical School Administration are underway and should be completed in the near future."

He added,

> I am extremely grateful to my many colleagues who were so helpful and considerate during the early period of establishment, growth, and development of the Section. I am indebted to my many friends on the faculty and in the administration of the Medical School at the University of Michigan. My special thanks go to Dr. C.G. Child, III who, in his careful and methodical manner, laid the groundwork and the solid foundation which eventuated in the official recognition of plastic surgery as a section of the Department of Surgery in the Medical School and the University Hospital. I also wish to express my thanks and appreciation to Dr. J.G. Turcotte who has maintained the high standards of the Department of Surgery.

It is with sadness and regret that I begin my terminal retirement furlough from the Department of Surgery and the Section of Plastic Surgery but it is with great pride and confidence that I turn over the reins to one of my illustrious former trainees, Dr. William C. Grabb. I am sure the section will have a bright future under his direction (Photo 31).[2]

Resident training and education were always in the forefront of Dr. Dingman's thoughts. In a 1968 *Plastic and Reconstructive Surgery (PRS) journal* article, he raised the question of how we are going to train enough plastic surgeons to provide care for the country's estimated population growth in the coming decades. At the time, there were only 725 board-certified plastic surgeons in the United States. One solution he offered was to shorten all aspects of the educational experience including one year less of K-12 and only three years of college premed. But more pertinent to our history here was his suggestion to shorten residency training as it existed at that time. Proposals included eliminating the internship and shortening prerequisite basic surgical training to three years, which would include exposure to all the related subspecialties, followed by two years of plastic surgery training with a third year optional. It is certainly conjecture, but the similarity is too close to ignore the possibility that these ideas in 1968 were the genesis of the 3 and 3 training program (discussed in detail in the following section "Dr. William C. Grabb's Tenure as Section Head") that was finally implemented in the section in 1973.

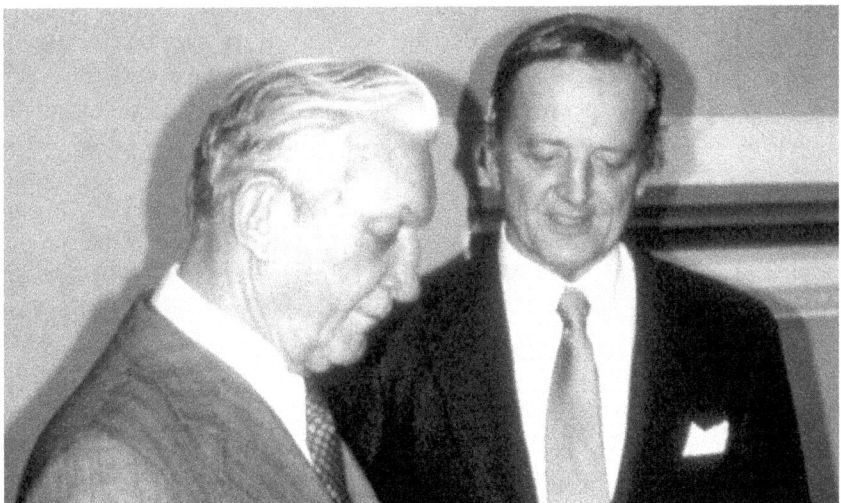

*Photo 31:* Drs. Dingman and Grabb at the time of transition in leadership.

To further improve the quality of the training experience, he felt that residents should be exposed to both clinical and laboratory research, that there should be exposure to preceptorship training experience, and that it was essential to teach surgical technique successfully enough to produce surgeons who could do superior plastic surgical operations. If not succeeding with the latter, he went on to say, "We have failed in our obligation as teachers of plastic surgeons."[3] As I look back, it appears that during Dr. Dingman's tenure, all these criteria were fulfilled as the section evolved under his exceptional leadership, in terms of the close surgical supervision provided in the operating room (OR), the preceptorship quality of the Saint Joseph Mercy Hospital (SJMH) rotation, the development of the laboratory program, and the continued interest of the faculty in clinical research. Although Dr. Dingman had retired as head of the section in 1975, he continued to be very active clinically and academically, maintaining a full operative schedule at SJMH and continuing to staff resident cases at the University of Michigan (UM). A retirement dinner in honor of Dr. Dingman was held in Ann Arbor in October of 1975 shortly after that year's American Society of Plastic and Reconstructive Surgery (ASPRS) meeting. In addition to his family and members of the UM plastic surgery family, a large number of his close professional friends and former trainees were in attendance.

## Dr. William C. Grabb's Tenure as Section Head

Dr. Grabb became temporary section head in July of 1975 and was officially appointed section head in 1976. Bill's wife, Cozy, told me recently that her recollection of this time was that from about 1973, Bill was being groomed for the leadership position in the section, taking on a lot of additional responsibilities.[4] He had already won several research awards, including the Robert H. Ivy award for best presentation of scientific material at the 1966 meeting of ASPRS and first prize in the essay contest from both the American Society for Surgery of the Hand (1968) and the Educational Foundation of ASPRS (1969). He had been president of the Educational Foundation (1973–74) and member of the Board of Directors of ASPRS, as well as associate editor of *PRS* starting in 1973. In addition, he had published the 1968 and 1973 editions of the very popular *Plastic Surgery—A Concise Guide to Clinical Practice*,[5] edited with his friend Jim Smith from New York City, which is still in print. This book was significant as it provided basic information about all aspects of the rapidly expanding field in an accessible form for both residents and medical students. In addition, Bill, with two other editors, edited *Cleft Lip and Palate: Surgical, Dental, and Speech Aspects* in 1971.[6] (For a full discussion of this book, see p. 95.)

Dr. Grabb, about 1973, with Dr. Dingman's strong endorsement, had instituted the "three-and-three" (3 and 3) resident training program and integrated it with the regular two-year residency program. This was the forerunner of the current integrated residency program, and subsequently, it was felt that Dr. Grabb was very prescient in introducing a program that would so significantly affect the future design of plastic surgery training. The applicants to this program were selected directly out of medical school and were highly regarded. They spent the first three years rotating through a variety of surgical specialties including some time on plastic surgery service at the university hospital. They were then integrated into the two-year formal plastic surgery residency and teamed with those residents who had completed their training in general surgery prior to entering the program. The 3 and 3 residents spent a sixth year of their training either in some combination with a laboratory research project or traveling to another training program in the United States or abroad. The mixture of these different levels of training and clinical expertise was a stimulant to all of us and enhanced the training experience positively. The residents who went through that program during that time included Larry Berkowitz, Glenn Harder, Roger Friedman, Rod Rohrich, Jeffrey Hamm, and Craig VanderKolk.

It was a small world in those days. Larry Berkowitz commented that he had the opportunity to be on the ENT service for six months because of Dr. Dingman's close relationship with Dr. Walter Work, the ENT department chair, who played poker with him every week. Larry shared his thoughts about the success of the 3 and 3 program: "If someone has a drive, a full course of general surgery may only serve to kill some of that enthusiasm. However, it does bring maturity, but that usually only comes with time, not necessarily training paths. I still feel a good plastic surgeon must start early and absorb as much from the various disciplines as possible to be a good problem solver."[7]

Medical student education was an early interest in the section and strongly supported by all three of us on the faculty. During those early years, we had four to five senior medical students at a time on a rotating surgical clerkship throughout the year. Using pigs' feet and commonly used plastic surgical instruments, we taught basic techniques for excising wounds and wound closure, and the technique of Z-plasty using various suture methods. In 1967, we published, in *PRS*, the details of the project and potential benefits experienced by a total of ninety students from the medical school classes of 1966 and 1967 who had rotated on the clerkship.[8] The exercise was considered quite useful by a wide majority of the students who were surveyed anonymously. Some of the students related the benefit to their actual patient care after graduation. Eventually, the required clerkship was discontinued, and it became an elective.

Consequently, we had fewer students on the service, but the teaching was continued on a case-by-case basis in the clinic and illustrated on patients in the OR.

Another important educational activity dear to Dr. Grabb's heart was the postgraduate course *Plastic Surgery in General Surgery Practice*. There were five biannual 2½-day conferences presented between 1969 and 1979 and designed for general surgeons and general practitioners (as family practice specialists were called in those days). The subjects covered were practical and focused on such techniques as skin grafting, best management of excising and repairing the defects after excising common skin lesions, and postmastectomy breast reconstruction. The courses were well attended and seemed to be very popular with attendees from around the state of Michigan as well as neighboring states. As an example (quoted from the section annual report 1971–72): "In 1971 there were 313 registered participants from 40 states. The great majority were general surgeons but other surgical specialties were represented."[9] It was noted in the annual report that this conference set an attendance record and the postgraduate education department agreed to sponsor it on a biennial basis. In addition to the UM plastic surgery faculty, Drs. Milton Edgerton (University of Virginia), Martin Entin (McGill), Frank Masters (University of Kansas), and John Simons (Mayo Clinic) participated along with additional UM faculty, Dr. Irving Feller (general surgery and head of Burn Center), Isadore Lampe (radiation therapy), and William Taylor (dermatology). Spreading the word about our current practices and new advances in plastic surgery helped to promote the activities of our new section and stimulated increased patient referrals.

One of the other projects for which I respected Dr. Grabb was the series of lectures he arranged for the entire staff on the techniques for interviewing patients. The lecturer was from the psychiatry department, and he stressed such aspects as not standing over a patient but sitting down before talking, not looking at the patient over the top of your glasses, and not taking notes (or I suppose nowadays not looking into a computer) but looking directly eye to eye with the patient. Most significantly, he stressed the importance of asking open-ended questions, not ones that could be answered by a single yes or no. Simple as it all sounds, these principles of interviewing were a revelation to many of us. The incorporation of these ideas served me well throughout my teaching experience and my own practice.

One of Bill's often-stated admonitions about patient evaluation for a physical problem was the importance of balancing the patient's concern in relation to the severity of whatever problem the patient presented. Dr. Mark Gorney, a well-known plastic surgeon, was one of Bill's good friends. He passed along to Bill the idea of using a graph that would

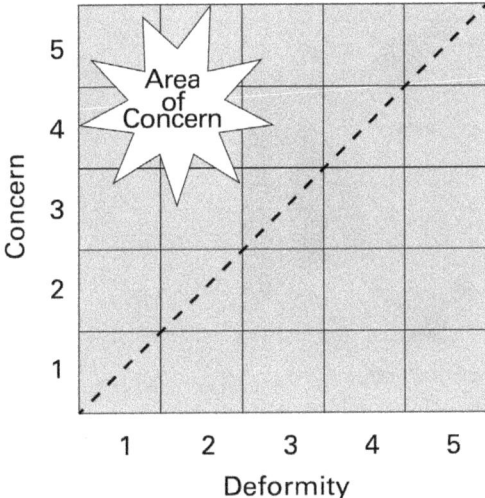

*Photo 32:* Graph depicting degree of severity of deformity (x axis) versus degree of patient's concern (y axis).

compare, in a straight-line relationship, a particular patient's aesthetic concern with the magnitude of the problem. Bill would often demonstrate the usefulness of such a graph in discussing a preoperative patient. Its use warned us to be wary when the patient's concern far exceeded the severity of the problem (see Photo 32). He encouraged all the residents to use this visual aid to help them evaluate patients' motivations and avoid an operation that would likely result in an unhappy and dissatisfied patient.

Dr. Grabb had played an important role in the initial training for the new Washtenaw County Emergency Medical Technician Training (EMT) program in the early and mid-1970s. The organizer was Jim Winkler, an SJMH general surgeon. Up until then, the only ambulance service in Ann Arbor was from the Staffan Funeral Home, located where the Campus Inn is now. Both Dr. Grabb and I gave lectures during the early training period. The graduates who had completed the EMT program as well as the physicians who were trained in the specialty of emergency care, which was subsequently developed, greatly enhanced the care of severely injured patients brought to the UM or SJMH emergency rooms.

During the subsequent years, Dr. Grabb continued to be a strong administrator, leader, and educator. The third edition of Grabb and Smith's *Plastic Surgery* was published in 1979. Grabb's book, *Skin Flaps*, edited with Bert Myers[10] (for details, see p. 76), was published in 1975 (discussed on pp. 77–9), while *Reconstruction and Rehabilitation of the Burned Patient*,[11] edited with Irving Feller was published in 1979. As if he

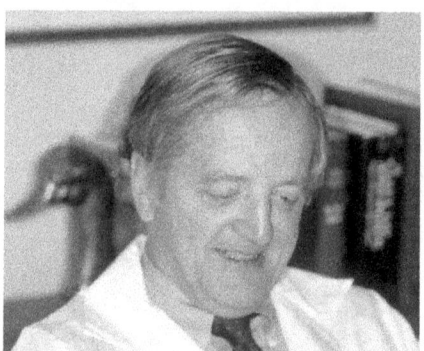
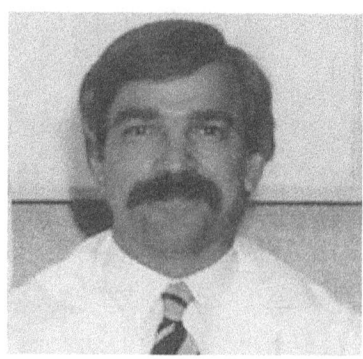

*Photo 33:* Dr. Grabb at his desk.

*Photo 34:* Dennis Bucko, MD.

were not busy enough during those years, he served as visiting professor at Cornell, University of Colorado, Johns Hopkins, walter Reed, George Washington University, and Universities of Baylor and Pennsylvania, as well as at programs in Caracas (in Venezuela) and Medellin (in Columbia).

Once Bill Grabb was established as head of the section, his leadership skills came to the fore. Something almost intangible was created by Bill in a very subtle, but effective, way. He was driven in his ambition but at the same time was extremely supportive to all his faculty. He always encouraged us in whatever direction we wanted to go and never put us down or criticized us in public. However, in private, he would kindly give us whatever advice he thought was necessary. He was one of those rare leaders who could make you feel better and more successful than you believed you deserved to be. By minimizing any tension as a result of competitiveness, he created an atmosphere of cooperation and fellowship that encouraged productivity, satisfaction, and happiness all at the same time. One other aspect of Bill Grabb's personality that served him well in his interpersonal academic relationships was his wonderful sense of humor. His willingness to project lightheartedness was often a welcome antidote when potential difficult or tense situations arose (Photo 33).

## Addition of New Faculty under Dr. Grabb's Leadership

Between 1976 and 1982, seven of the new alumni of the UM training program were asked to stay on as new faculty members.

**Dr. Dennis Bucko** stayed on in Ann Arbor after he finished his residency in 1976 at the UM. He was appointed instructor in plastic surgery with a 50 percent appointment (Photo 34). He saw his private patients at Dr. Dingman's office. This was right around the time that Dr. Dingman retired as section head. Bill Grabb had moved his office from the Ingalls Street location to the university hospital as he was in transition to becoming permanent head of the section. Dr. Bucko was appointed to the medical staff at SJMH, and his private patients were hospitalized there. Right after he finished his training, he spent two to three weeks in New York City with Byron Smith and his oculoplastic team. He also spent some time with Dr. John M. Converse. When he returned to Ann Arbor, he started evaluating oculoplastic patients in the plastic surgery clinic at the university hospital and assumed teaching assignments with ophthalmology residents. This fit well with Dr. Grabb's idea that the faculty should each try to gain special expertise in some aspect of plastic surgery.

Dennis was following a family with more than one child who had congenital absence of upper eyelid levator muscles. He treated them surgically with silicon slings to replace the levator function. He also covered the pediatric residents at Mott Hospital and did quite a bit of hand surgery and general plastic surgery in private practice at SJMH. Dennis made significant contributions in teaching the residents many aspects of plastic surgery and nerve grafting in primates in the lab (see p. 64 for details). We were all sorry to see Dennis leave Ann Arbor in 1981 to start a private practice in southern California. He was well liked and had made significant contributions to the teaching program.

**Dr. M. Haskell (Hack) Newman** finished his two years of plastic surgery training at the UM in 1977 (Photo 35). Hack's previous training included completing an otolaryngology residency in 1968 at UM with a master of science degree in acoustic physiology. After a tour in the army, he joined the faculty at the UM and became an assistant professor in the Department of Otolaryngology until 1975. Just prior to starting his plastic surgery residency, he completed a fellowship in facial plastic surgery with Dr. Richard Webster in Boston. Then for the first six months after completing his training in plastic surgery in June of 1977, he took a craniofacial (CF) fellowship in Toronto, Canada, with Dr. Ian Munro. When he returned to Ann Arbor, Hack assumed a full-time academic position as assistant professor in plastic surgery and established an office on Clark Road near SJMH, where he became a member of the medical staff and hospitalized his private patients. He was active in teaching residents at the UM and passed on much important information to all of us, both faculty and residents, about rhinoplasty and other aesthetic procedures that he had

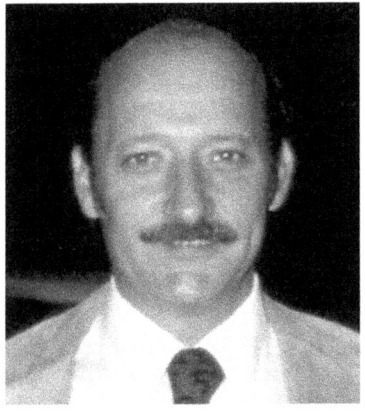

Photo 35: M. Haskell Newman, MD.

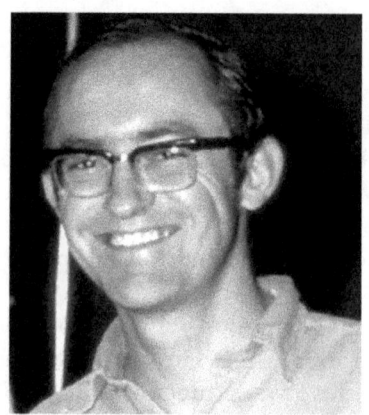

Photo 36: Louis Mes, MD.

learned in his previous ENT career and from his time with Dr. Webster. He also was the primary staff member at the Ann Arbor Veterans Administration (VA) Hospital (part of the university hospital system) for resident training during that time. In 1981, he shifted his responsibilities to half-time at the university and moved his office to the Reichert Health Building, attached to SJMH. He continued covering the resident service at the VA Hospital and the pediatric service at Mott Hospital. Returning from Toronto, he was able to get the CF program underway together with neurosurgery (see pp. 117–9). He was aided by Dr. Eddie Kahn, previous head of neurosurgery, who was still active clinically. Together with Dr. Louis Argenta, the two were able to expand the CF service to both adults and children.

**Dr. Louis Mes** stayed on the faculty as an instructor for a year after completing the residency in 1977 (Photo 36). This is the story of how that came about in Dr. Mes's own words:

> I wanted to go back to South Africa (SA) and for that matter my J1 visa demanded it, but there was a technical glitch with the SA licensing board over my title during my spell in Scotland and they wanted three more months of accredited training on my CV before I could practice in SA. Getting a residency in SA to do just three months was almost impossible and they wanted me to re-do my whole residency in SA. This was ridiculous, so Bill Grabb created a job for me at the "U" and I stayed on for a year as a clinical instructor to solve the problem.

This is a good example of Bill's generosity in helping his residents and the trust the residents had in Bill. Continuing in Dr. Mes's words,

> I had been doing a research project on manipulating cell metabolism with steroids and allopurinol to improve graft and flap survival, and was able to complete the work during that year. The Department of Surgery awarded me the Coller Prize for original research at the annual Senior Residents meeting for my paper, and it was later published in *PRS*. My job as clinical instructor involved staffing the residents at Jackson Prison and most of it was done with Paul Dempsey and later with Eric Austad. The experience we all received working there stands me in great stead, even today.[12]

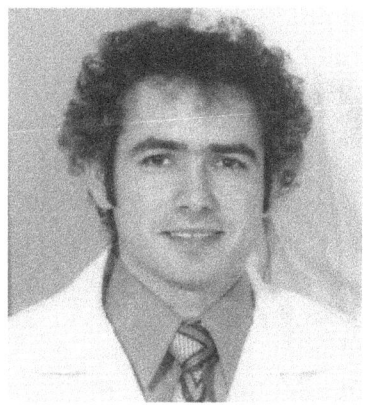
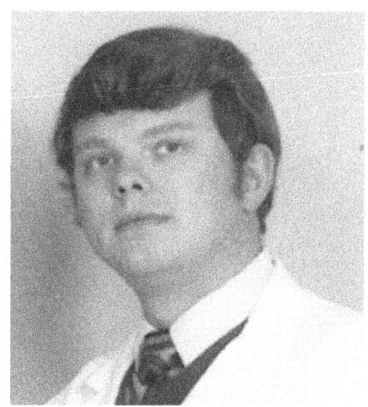

Photo 37: Paul H. Izenberg, MD.

Photo 38: Eric Austad, MD.

**Dr. Paul H. Izenberg** completed the UM residency in 1978 and joined John Markley and me in our practice at the Tower Plaza (Photo 37). Paul had many other opportunities to practice but really wanted to stay in Ann Arbor. Thus, he followed Dr. Dingman's remembered admonition, "Don't stay here just because you are afraid to go somewhere else."[13] He was appointed to the faculty as an instructor in plastic surgery. There will always appear some stresses and strains when a new faculty member joins a program, especially in a small group as we were then. However, they were short-lived. Paul rapidly became a welcome and essential addition to the program because of his surgical skills, artistic talent, and creative ability to innovate. It is interesting and gratifying to see how much collegiality quickly developed and was maintained among the faculty then and in subsequent years. I believe that these feelings of respect and friendship greatly enhanced the success of the residency program overall.

**Dr. Eric D. Austad** also finished his residency in 1978 (Photo 38). Following this, he received a half-time appointment as clinical instructor at UM and continued his work on skin expansion in the Sargent plastic surgery laboratory. He also provided faculty coverage for plastic residents on clinical rotation to Jackson Prison for 1½ years. During that period, he was also on staff at Henry Ford plastic surgery service. In 1981, he started practice at Chelsea Hospital and began consulting about specific head and neck nerves associated with intractable headache problems in collaboration with Dr. Saper and others in their neurology group who specialized in headache management. In 1983, he joined Hack Newman in practice at SJMH with an office in the Reichert Health Building and continued his teaching and research in skin expansion as clinical assistant professor.

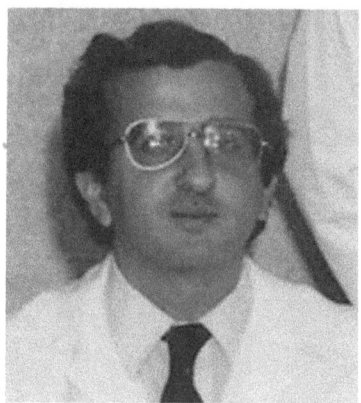 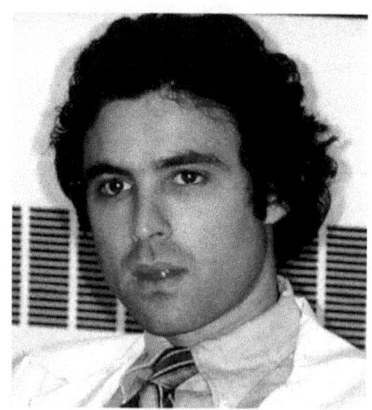

Photo 39: Louis Argenta, MD.   Photo 40: Malcolm Marks, MD.

**Dr. Louis C. Argenta (Lou)** finished his plastic surgery training in 1979 (Photo 39). He was only the third resident in the program who, prior to plastic surgery residency, had completed a full general surgery residency at UM. All the others were in the 3 and 3 program or had prior training at other institutions. He then went to Paris for several months to study with Dr. Paul Tessier, a world famous CF surgeon. He returned to UM as assistant professor and took on many teaching responsibilities. After Dr. Grabb's death, Lou, as a very essential member of the faculty, took over many important administrative responsibilities. Clinically, in addition to other duties, he helped Hack Newman further develop the CF program.

**Dr. Malcolm Marks** was a resident from 1980 to 1982, and after four months of travel at the end of his residency, he spent a year in the Sargent laboratory working with Dr. Mike Morykwas (Photo 40). He spent that year researching the effect of mechanical deformation of soft tissues, particularly blood flow using radioactive microspheres and tissue oxygen level in response to skin expansion. His activities on the faculty when he returned are discussed in the Epilogue (p. 146).

## Dr. Grabb's Unexpected Death and Subsequent Events

In 1982, Dr. Grabb's sudden, unexpected death was a devastating blow to the section and to everyone associated with plastic surgery at the UM. It was especially hard on the residents who were in the midst of their training. Dr. Robert Gilman (resident, 1980–82) has recounted this period very accurately:

> I was sitting there deep in conversation with L3 around 5 pm on a March afternoon in 1982 when Dr. Grabb emerged from his office

holding a wicker basket by its handle, filled with a manuscript of his latest book project, "The Encyclopedia of Flaps." He was excited to be leaving on a "working" vacation to his home on Man O War Key in the Bahamas. From my seat by the door I watched him walk down the hall toward the elevators. This was the last time I or, for that matter, anyone from Plastic Surgery at the University of Michigan saw Dr Grabb.[14]

Lauralee recollected well what happened next: "Dr. Oneal (having learned the tragic news from Mrs. Grabb) phoned me at home on the evening of March 31, 1982 to tell me that Dr. Grabb had died while on vacation in the Bahamas. He then asked me to notify the residents so I phoned Bob Gilman, a senior resident, and asked him to spread the word."[15] Dr. Gilman continued,

It was early Sunday evening when I received a call on my home phone from L3 telling me to brace myself for some awful news. Dr. William C. Grabb, the Head of our Plastic Surgery program at the University of Michigan, had died suddenly and unexpectedly while jogging on Man O War Key. He had gone out for a jog and when he didn't return a search for him by the local authorities discovered his body on the jogging path. L3 asked me to contact all my fellow residents. I remember the disbelief, confusion, and fear we all shared. Fortunately, Dr. Dingman quickly agreed to come back as interim Head bringing some stability back to the program.[16]

Lauralee recollected, "The next day at work was unreal as the shocking news traveled fast. The phone rang constantly with the same question asked every time: 'Is it true?' Yes, sadly it was true."[17] "Dr. Dingman was soon appointed as Acting or Interim Head of the Section and he returned to a familiar leadership role. His very presence was calming as he was always our anchor."[18]

Dr. Gilman continued, "Our graduation certificates were signed by Dr. Dingman. The memorial service for Dr. Grabb was somber and attended by many notable Plastic Surgeons from around the country. Many former residents came back to Ann Arbor for the service."[19] Dr. Malcolm Marks, who was a resident with Dr. Gilman, recalled, "Dr. Grabb gave me my start in plastic surgery. He accepted me into one of the finest programs in the country where he maintained an academic atmosphere while prompting the importance of a busy clinical environment. His intellect, love of academic medicine, and teaching while being a busy clinician inspired the professional goals I have tried to emulate."[20]

Dr. Dingman, in a eulogy to Bill, created a verbal portrait that embodies so many of Bill's outstanding personal, leadership, and academic qualities. Quoting in part,

> As I reflect upon the life and accomplishments of Bill Grabb, I recognize that he was a person of great self-discipline. He set realistic goals and objectives for himself, and had the ability to plan a course that would lead to their achievement. For each event he would develop a plan, write a scenario, set a timetable, and work doggedly toward completion on schedule. He so organized his life that he allocated definite periods each week to work on various projects. Sometimes he could be found in a carrel in the medical center library, or in the anatomy laboratory, or in the animal operating room in the Kresge Research Center. It was these work habits, supplemented by long hours in his study at home, and even on his frequent journeys to his beloved island, that led to significant research on unsolved problems in plastic and reconstructive surgery. This also includes his four textbooks, publication of over 60 scientific articles, and preparation of another textbook he was working on at the time of his death. He made literally hundreds of presentations at local, national, and international meetings. Bill had the unique ability to conceptualize scientific meetings and congresses two or three years in advance, and to work diligently to attract international authorities to participate in topic discussions at these educational forums. He also had the ability to enlist the aid of colleagues in these events and tactfully make constructive suggestions to those who willingly agreed to participate. This is demonstrated most vividly by his ability to get 60–80 plastic surgery authorities to compile textbooks with him. Bill Grabb was a master of organization, not only in achieving his own goals, but in the administration of the Section of Plastic Surgery at the University of Michigan where everyone had an assignment and was expected to carry it out with dispatch and on time. He expected no more of others than he himself could do or had already done. But he did require every one of his colleagues and associates to reach for perfection and "carry the message to Garcia." One of Bill's favorite quotations was from this great philosophical tract of Elbert Hubbard, and I quote: "the world cries out for such: he is needed, and needed badly—the man who can carry a message to Garcia." If you are not acquainted with this literary work, I would urge you to go and read it. You will then understand Bill Grabb better and you will know why I now (close) by saying—Bill Grabb has succeeded. He has taken his message

to Garcia, and now on to Heaven.[21] (For a citation of Hubbard's book and a description of it, see A-12 in the appendix. Also see the appendix for memorial comments from the six residents in training when Dr. Grabb died.)

Lauralee again related what followed:

> My own work concentrated on notifying people of Dr. Grabb's death and writing obituaries. Somehow we comforted each other while grieving in private. Dr. Louis Argenta, a close colleague of Dr. Grabb, worked with Dr Dingman to keep the Section running. Coverage still had to be provided for the E.R., O.R., clinics, and referrals. A high degree of normalcy was the goal, and Drs. Argenta and Dingman achieved it well with full cooperation from all the staff and residents. The value of Dr. Dingman being available and capable during this time should be thoroughly appreciated. I believe that he literally saved the Section of Plastic Surgery as no one else could have done, reducing recovery time by months.[22]

Another acknowledgment was stated in a letter to Dr. Dingman from Dr. Oneal: "I wanted to take this opportunity to formally thank you, from the bottom of my heart, for all the effort you have made on our collective behalf during your tenure as acting head. It has been an extraordinary experience for all of us. Had you not been willing to step into the breach, I think we all would have suffered. There is no question that your taking over as acting head has given all of us the strength to maintain a first class program." Dr. Malcolm Marks recounted his impressions of Dr. Dingman: "By the time I had the honor and good fortune of meeting Dr. Dingman, he was 74 years old and towards the end of his career. I was aware of his professional achievements and he was a legend to a young surgeon. I was astounded by the power, strength, and stamina of a man that age. It made me wish I had seen him just for a moment in his youth."[23]

In the early 1980s, Dr. Grabb had made it clear that he wanted to increase the number of full-time faculty members. He was seeking someone with clinical skills as well as laboratory experience. Josh Jurkiewicz, head of the highly respected plastic surgery training program at Emory University in Atlanta, proposed one of his graduating trainees, Dr. Tom Stevenson (see Group Photo 1983). For Dr. Grabb, Tom was the perfect fit, and it was arranged that he would join the faculty in July 1982. Even after Dr. Grabb's untimely death in March of that year, Dr. Stevenson agreed to fulfill his commitment, and he arrived in Ann Arbor as scheduled. In addition to being well trained in all aspects of plastic surgery, he brought knowledge and skills concerning myocutaneous flaps, microvascular surgery, and treatment of long-bone osteomyelitis. He had an inquiring mind, was a good teacher, and immediately became an essential member of the section.

From 1982 to 1984, the program continued to thrive under Dr. Dingman's strong leadership. In addition, during this time, a search committee was formed to seek a new permanent head of the section. The selection process ended with Dr. Jeremiah Turcotte, chairman of the surgery department, appointing Dr. Steve Mathes, a very well-known and highly respected clinical and research surgeon, as section head in 1984 (see Group Photo 1985). Dr. Mathes left after one year and returned to California to become head of plastic surgery at the University of California, San Francisco (UCSF). Dr. Louis Argenta was appointed interim section head by Dr. Turcotte, and another search committee was formed. Dr. Argenta had been engaged in a wide range of clinical activities in collaboration with Dr. Dingman and Dr. Malcolm Marks beyond the CF program already mentioned in Dr. Newman's resume. The work of Drs. Marks and Argenta is discussed in greater detail in the chapter seven as well as in the epilogue.

CHAPTER FIVE

# Early Clinical Rotations and Teaching Conferences

During most of the term of Dr. Dingman's (ROD) tenure as section head, the resident rotations and defined responsibilities took the following form:

*Junior resident (first year).* There were three periods of four months each: plastic surgery (PS) service at University of Michigan Hospital (UMH), PS service at Saint Joseph Mercy Hospital (SJMH), and hand surgery rotation in Detroit. Their duties, especially at UMH and SJMH, included pre-post-op care, assisting in all surgical procedures of the service, ward rounds at least twice a day, wound care, and dressing changes. They also had to staff the outpatient clinic four days a week, attend all plastic surgery conferences, maintain photography files, and perform independent operative procedures under direct supervision of faculty and/or a senior (second-year) resident.

*Senior resident.* Senior residents also rotated through three periods of four months each: adult PS service at UMH and pediatric PS service at the new Mott Hospital. Rotations also included the Ann Arbor Veterans Administration Hospital (VA), Wayne County General Hospital (WCGH), and the Southern Michigan State Prison (Jackson Prison). Duties included performing increased numbers of independent operative procedures under staff supervision, in addition to assuming primary responsibility for care of patients on the wards and outpatient clinics; teaching junior residents, interns, and medical students; and attending all conferences, patient rounds, and weekly meetings. They were also encouraged to complete any clinical or laboratory research projects they had started.

Initially, in the rotation schedule, there was a three-month rotation for the junior residents on the newly formed UM Burn Unit. However, almost all of the residents in the first years of the university program had completed general surgery and felt they had ample experience in the acute care of burns. The rotation was stressful for some of them. Ted Dodenhoff (1967–69) recollected, "My first rotation was to the Burn Unit and no two people in the world clashed more than Irv Feller (general surgeon who ran the Burn Unit) and me. I was close to getting thrown out when Dr. Dingman took me aside and pointed out that I was giving up my future if I didn't suck it up and get through the next three months. I did and he was right. If he hadn't taken a personal interest in me, my bullheadedness would have been the end of me."[1] This was a good example of the personal interest Dr. Dingman took in all his residents. The staff soon after decided to terminate residents' rotation on the Burn Unit. We realized that our residents, fully trained surgeons, had already received adequate training in the acute care of burn patients. The PS service continued to be involved in the care of secondary burn deformities.

## Resident Rotations at Saint Joseph Mercy Hospital

Resident rotations at SJMH were, from the beginning, an important part of the plastic surgery training program, as all of Dr. Dingman's, Dr. Grabb's, and my private patients had their operations there. Two residents rotated on this service, usually a first-year resident and often a resident rotating from Ford Hospital for six months. Sometimes, there was also a fellow. Dr. Isaac Peled was a fellow for a year in 1976–77. He remembers Dr. Dingman's pace quite well: "We operated at SJMH from 7 AM to whatever it takes and from there to the clinic until evening. I was on my feet at 5 AM and when we finished the clinic ROD sometimes said, 'OK boys you can take the rest of the day off, we'll meet at 7 a.m.'"[2] There was a great variety of patients on the service who enhanced the training experience. In the operating room (OR), Dr. Dingman trusted the residents and gave them a tremendous amount of responsibility in preparing the patients for surgery, marking for reductions, anesthetizing the nose for rhinoplasty, and properly prepping and draping the patient. When he walked into the OR, he expected to start the procedure without delay. It was somewhat nerve-wracking for the resident, but a great training experience. Dr. Ernie Manders's personal memory illustrates the tremendous influence Dr. Dingman had on his residents: "The St. Joe rotation was a busy one and my first time to really work with Dr. Dingman. Few men whom I have met have equaled him in inspiring memories filled with admiration. He was a hard worker but never too busy to teach. He was generous and gracious to everyone. He was looking ahead and fiercely in pursuit of excellence in all things. And working with him, he let you into his luminous life."[3] In addition to the many innovations that he developed, we especially admired his open-mindedness to new ideas. An example was in 1966 when, as a senior resident at SJMH and working with Dr. Harvey Weiss who was rotating from Ford Hospital, I had read an article about treatment of congenital cup ear by expansion of the helical cartilage that Dr. Dingman had not seen as yet. It was written by Dr. Ross Musgrave, a good friend of his from Pittsburgh.[4] I brought the article into the OR because we had a case that morning of a young patient with exactly that deformity. When Dr. Dingman arrived in the OR, I showed him the article, and he said that it looked like a good idea and might be a significant improvement on current techniques. So we followed the technique that Dr. Musgrave had described and the patient had an excellent result. Bob Wilensky (resident, 1973–75) related that "his last rotation in medical school at U of M was on private plastic surgery service at SJMH and the residents were Bob Oneal and Harvey Weiss. When he returned to the program seven years later in 1973 as a resident, Wilensky noted that Dr. Dingman had modified virtually every operation he was doing from how he had done it in the 1960s."[5] This is another example of how Dr. Dingman was always adapting, growing, and trying to keep up to date with the latest and best operations available.

Another important part of the training program occurred at Dr. Dingman's office located across Ingalls Street from SJMH where he, Dr. Grabb, and I (for three years) saw private patients together with the residents assigned to SJMH (Photo 41). On Tuesdays and Thursdays, Dr. Ding-

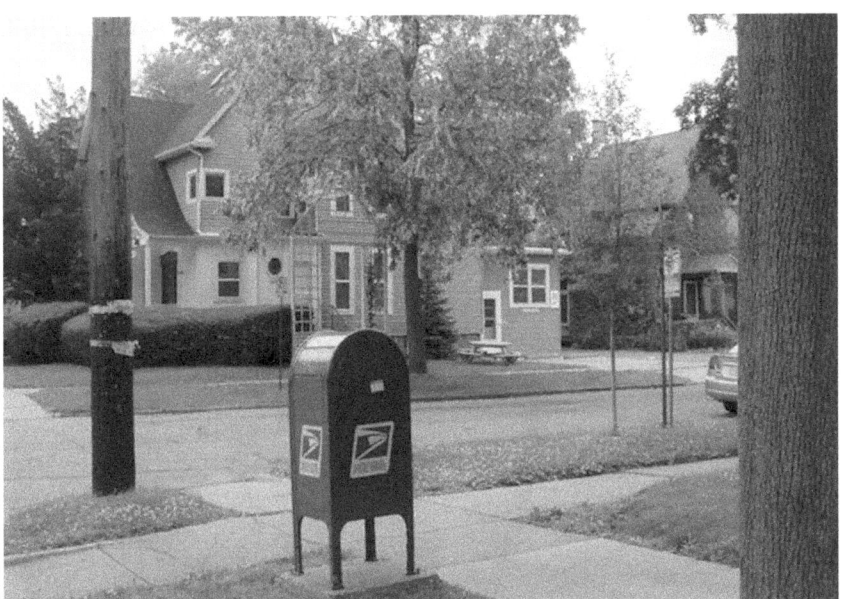

*Photo 41:* Drs. Dingman and Grabb's Ingalls Street office with mailbox across Catherine Street in the foreground.

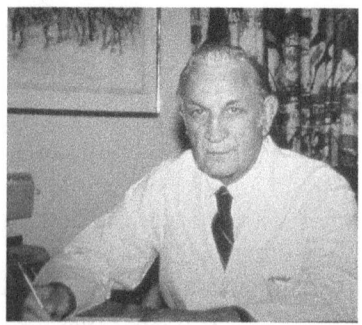

*Photo 42:* Dr. Dingman in his private office across Ingalls Street.

man operated at the university. On Mondays, Wednesdays, and Fridays, he operated at SJMH. On those days, he would arrive at his office to see patients when he had finished his two or three cases and rounds (Photo 42). By the time he arrived, the number of waiting office patients would have often spilled out onto the lawn and sidewalk in front of the private office. Sometimes, office hours ran from 5:00 p.m. to 11:00 p.m. There was always tea and snacks on Dr. Dingman's desk, and smoking was not allowed except in the basement. At the end of office hours, Mrs. Schilling, the office manager, expected the residents to take the office mail to a mailbox across the street from the Ingalls Street office on their way back to SJMH. She was a formidable presence, ran a tight ship, and was very efficient and much loved by Dr. Dingman. In the basement of the office, there were large illuminated sliding files of 35 mm slides of pre- and post-op as well as operative views of patients with all varieties of conditions and who had undergone various procedures, which were collected over many years. They were a wonderful educational resource. Dr. Dingman was very proud of his camera setup with a double light source designed to avoid shadows. He carried it with him in a case along with the "Dingman Blue" wool background and used it for all patient-related photographs (see Photo 43).

*Photo 43:* Dr. Dingman's 35 mm camera setup with the double flash system. On a plaque on the case for the camera, now kept in the Plastic Surgery Clinic, is a statement from Dr. Turcotte to whom Dr. Dingman, at his retirement, gave the camera. It states that Dr. Dingman was "dedicated to promoting and improving medical photography. For many years he set the standard for the entire surgical staff at Michigan."

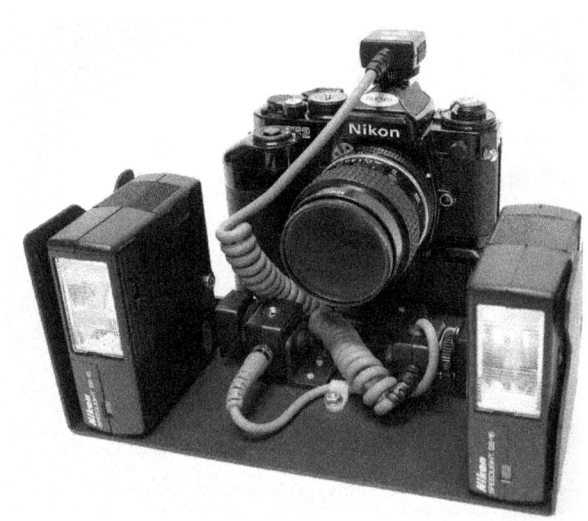

In those days, almost all plastic surgery patients, including aesthetic and hand surgery patients who were to be operated on, had to be admitted preoperatively the night before. So a patient getting operated on Monday would get admitted on Sunday. This meant Sunday afternoon/evening rounds with Dr. Dingman often cut into the residents' family time. Dr. Dingman expected his residents to be available on quick notice as Ted Dodenhoff remembered: "The thing I remember the most were those calls from the airport (from ROD): Ted, just got back in town and I'd like to meet you on the ward in 45 minutes for rounds."[6]

A few selected patients were brought in by a family member or a friend the "same day" for procedures such as blepharoplasty or other special cases. At home, they would take 200 mg of Seconal (secobarbital), and when they arrived in the preoperative area, they would get Demerol before their local anesthetic. This combination served as their preoperative sedation before the days of Valium (diazepam) and Xanax (alprazolam). That was the early form of same-day surgery, but it was pretty primitive to say the least. As we had no facility or staff outside of the hospital for monitoring our patients postoperatively, they would stay at least overnight or sometimes a few nights depending on which procedure they had undergone.

At the time, most of the emergency and elective hand surgery at SJMH was being handled by our plastic surgical staff and so the residents on rotation there were exposed to a fair amount of hand surgery experience. After 1975, one of the residents on rotation at SJMH was assigned to Dr. Markley, who provided a very thorough tutorial in hand surgery in the OR, reviewing office patients, and with weekly one-on-one seminars.

At that time, in addition to our private patients, all three of us, Drs. Oneal, Markley, and Izenberg (OMI), were covering the residents' cases at the university hospital OR or one of the clinics at least one or two days per week up until 1984. Our office was still located in the Tower Plaza that we loved due to its downtown location and proximity to the old SJMH hospital. We remained there even after SJMH relocated between 1975 and 1977 from Ingalls Street to its present location on East Huron River Drive (see Photo 44). However, by 1977, it was clear that the distance to our hospital patients and the emergency room at SJMH was a hindrance to our availability and good patient care. Dr. Izenberg first, and then Dr. Markley and I, moved to a new office on Clark Road near SJMH.

Before 1979, most of the outpatient cosmetic surgeries were performed at Saline or Chelsea Hospital, and the patients were admitted overnight. About 1980, at SJMH, we (OMI) began performing some outpatient aesthetic surgery in our office. Dr. Izenberg gave the IV sedation for the first couple of cases of augmentations. We then hired a group of well-trained and excellent certified registered nurse anesthetists (CRNAs), Jeanne Learman, Donna Smith, and LuAnn Stencil. We were very happy

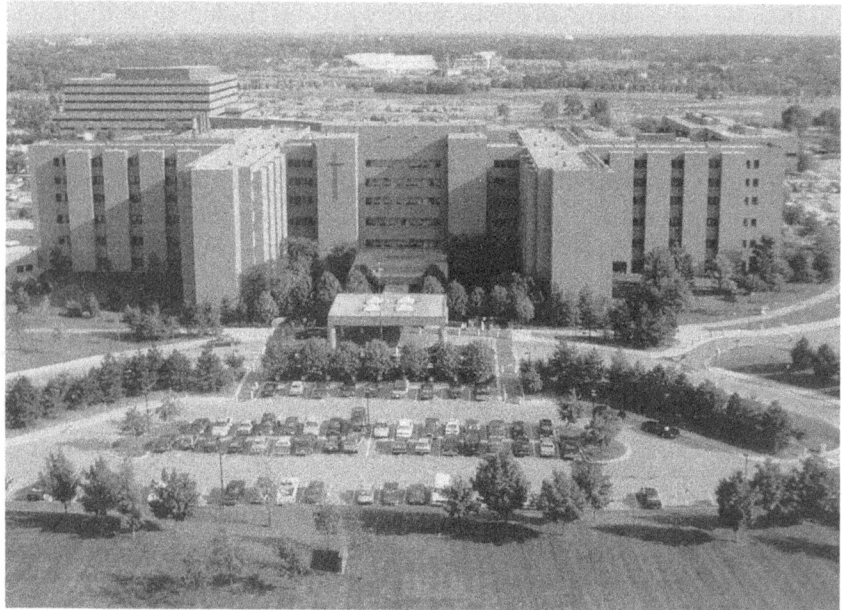

*Photo 44:* New (now old) SJMH on Huron River Drive east of Ann Arbor (c. 1977).

with their expertise and the increased patient safety they provided. The eventual availability of short-acting sedation agents facilitated better utilization of our office OR and contributed to the success of the practice and convenience for our patients. This was also a good experience for the residents as this was about the only outpatient surgery experience they had until the opening of an ambulatory surgical facility (ASF) at SJMH. Dr. Malcolm Marks recently told me his thoughts about his experience as a resident at SJMH in 1981: "When I think back on my education I remember how critical the experience was at St. Joes. The full- and part-time faculty demonstrated that however important it is to provide the best care to a patient it is not enough. They all demonstrated their love of their profession and dedication to passing their skills on to upcoming generations. Each taught not by just imparting their knowledge and skill in the OR and conferences, but by example. They repeatedly demonstrated their intellectual curiosity and concern for patient and resident education."[7]

## Rotations at University of Michigan Hospital

There were usually both a first-year and a second-year resident rotating on this service and occasionally one of the fellows. In the early period, almost all the patients were considered resident cases with staff coverage. After becoming section head in 1975, Dr. Grabb operated on his private patients at the university. However, there were clearly delineated resident cases staffed by all members of the faculty on a rotating basis. All of us on the faculty had assigned days to cover both the OR and the clinic. Until Mott Hospital was built, adults and children were operated on in the main hospital. However, during those years, the most outstanding benefit for the residents was assisting Dr. Dingman with his private patients at SJMH and operating with his assistance at the university hospital. As trainees, all the residents admired and respected Dr. Dingman a great deal, particularly for his commitment to excellence in all aspects of plastic surgery, including surgical skill, care for patients, thoughtful and kind personal relationships with colleagues and staff, and an emphasis on the clarity of photographic documentation.

All trainees in the early years of the program tried to emulate Dr. Dingman, and in return, he was very proud of all those he trained. The following quotation from Grant Fairbanks (1969–71), I believe, reflects the feelings of all the residents: "Although his residents were all fully trained general surgeons, Dr. Dingman taught us the finer points about the art of medicine, dealing with private patients in the clinic, taking patient photographs, record keeping, correspondence with colleagues, and other important items. He would frequently dictate his clinical notes in the patient's room in front of the patient. What characterized Dr. Dingman above all else was that he was 'always a gentleman' in every situation."[8]

In 1969, the original Mott Children's Hospital opened and replaced the pediatric wards at the "old main" university hospital. The PS service was offered the opportunity to move not only its pediatric patients to the new facility but also all its adult patients to a separate unit. Except for a few extremely complicated cases, all the operations were also done in the new ORs in Mott. This helped fill the beds in the new hospital but also was an upgrade for our adult patients who were now in double rooms instead of the eighteen-bed wards in the "old main." The resident coverage was then split into pediatric and adult services. When the new university hospital opened in 1986, our adult patients were moved there. Sometime before that, the Taubman Outpatient Building opened in its current location. Our clinical offices, exam rooms, and secretaries moved into quarters on the second floor of the new outpatient building, which was directly connected to the soon-to-be-opened new main hospital.

## Hand Rotation in Detroit

The hand surgery service at old Grace Hospital in Detroit, Michigan, was under the direction of Dr. Joseph Posch, assisted by Drs. Robert

Larsen, Eugene Harrell, and Kim Lie. Dr. Don Davis recalled, "We all went there for three months and it was an important and gratifying experience for the majority of us."[9] The UM residents shared the rotation with residents from Duke University. It was a busy service with often three to four hand cases a day of great variety on the operating schedule. Frequently, as many as one hundred pre- and post-op patients would be seen in the office in a single day. It was a wonderful introduction to hand surgery as our residents were exposed to a wide range of ideas. One of these ideas, to be specific, was a technique of placing a periosteal flap over the fresh-cut surface of a revision on an amputated phalanx. Dr. Larsen had been using this technique for some time, and he was convinced that it led to less post-op pain at the amputation site. So we wrote it up and I presented it at the American Society of Plastic and Reconstructive Surgery (ASPRS), and it was published in *the Plastic and Reconstructive Surgery journal* in 1966.[10] In subsequent years, the group of attendings in the Detroit practice split, and our residents were assigned to Dr. Larsen, who, according to Paul Izenberg on his rotation to Detroit, was a workaholic in addition to being an excellent surgeon. At Paul's time, the rotation included a daily schedule of five to six hours in the OR, repairing the results of factory-induced hand injuries. This was followed by office hours sometimes running for five to six hours into the evening. Paul related a fascinating aspect of the experience at Old Grace Hospital:

> I do remember one "spooky" thing. When we stayed in Detroit while on call, the assigned sleeping room was located in the old Grace Hospital, no longer used but still attached to the new Harper-Grace where we operated. The corridors were dark and the ceilings very high. It was always chilly and not a soul was around. I was told the room we stayed in was Houdini's when he became sick while performing in Detroit. He actually died in that very room on October 31, 1928 (Halloween). I didn't realize that a séance had been held there every year on the anniversary of his death by his fans trying to make contact with him. That made it even more of a creepy place to stay and, as you can imagine, I didn't get much rest.[11]

Shortly after Paul's junior residency year in 1977, John Markley had established a solid hand tutorial program in Ann Arbor, and the Detroit hand rotation was eventually discontinued. The time with these excellent hand surgeons had provided a much welcome experience in hand surgery for the resident training during those preceding fourteen years.

## Wayne County General Hospital Rotation

This hospital was located in Westland, Michigan, about ten miles east of Ann Arbor. It was a large general hospital, and the UM orthopedic and gynecological surgery residents who rotated there got a tremendous amount of surgical experience as did our residents. Early on, Bill Grabb and I were the staff physicians covering the plastic surgery patients. Our plastic surgery residents rotated there on a regular basis, had a lot of independence, and did a lot of cases. When Dr. Markley joined the faculty, he took over covering the service, followed by Dr. Bucko, and was eventually replaced by Dr. Izenberg after he joined the faculty. WCGH was closed as a result of a decision by the county administration in 1984. Dr. Izenberg recalls his experience there as a young faculty member:

> A few thoughts on the Wayne County General Hospital on Merriman Road just north of the Detroit airport. The junior resident ran an independent plastic surgery service at Wayne County with weekly clinics and block OR time. As you can imagine, most of the patients were trauma (auto and gunshot) or brought in from the long-term psychiatric facility attached to the hospital by a long tunnel. Pressure sores, facial fractures, some burns, breast reductions, and general trauma were the daily fare. Occasionally we saw a cosmetic case. It was a good rotation for residents as they had full patient responsibility assisted by an assigned attending. I was fortunate enough to take this over after Dennis Bucko moved on. I found it a good opportunity to work closely one on one with the residents but giving them the freedom to make their own decisions. There certainly were some tough actors (patients) out there like motorcycle gangs. There was the story that rival motorcycle gangs had driven in to the ER and tore it up a year or two before I arrived for my internship in 1969. So we had plenty of armed guards (not as many as the Jackson Prison rotation!). Although the drive was tough in the winter, the rotation was a good learning experience and a shame that it went away in the late 1980s.[12]

## Jackson Prison Rotation

The State Prison at Jackson, Michigan, about forty miles west of Ann Arbor, may be the largest walled prison in the world. The focus of plastic surgical care at Jackson Prison was rehabilitating the prisoners who were to be released or to be put on parole so they might experience reduced recidivism. After years of prison life, many inmates experience extremely low self-esteem related to their appearance. They fear that they will be labeled as an "ex-con" and will have little chance of being accepted in the outside world. This was the stimulus for plastic surgery involvement. Even though the initial emphasis was on scar revisions and tattoo removals, Dr. Mes recalls that a wide variety of procedures were undertaken[13]: hair transplants, face-lifts, rhinoplasties, and total ear and nasal reconstructions were among the many other procedures that were felt might be helpful. As both Drs. Berner and Manders recalled, all of the residents in the program spent time on a regular schedule in both the plastic surgery clinic and the OR. They both recalled that there was a grant from the State of Michigan to support this rehabilitation program.[14,15]

At the beginning, those of us on the faculty rotated staff coverage, but the senior residents were allowed a significant amount of independence. Dr. Fairbanks remembered Dr. Dingman coming out to the prison to assist with rhinoplasties. He recounted doing twenty-one rhinoplasties with Dr. Dingman's assistance. He stated that the prison program was an important part of the residency as the caseload was high while also providing experience in a wide variety of procedures.[16] Later, Drs. Mes and Austad assumed the faculty staffing responsibilities. The prisoners developed respect and friendship with these young, caring surgeons. An example is well documented by Dr. Carl Berner (resident, 1969–71):

> I had the opportunity to help rehabilitate an "amazing" inmate. As a young man, he killed a teller in a bank robbery. He avoided arrest for several months and was on the list of the ten most wanted. He sought "help" from a "surgeon" in Canada in an effort to change his appearance. Under sedation his surgeon flattened his nose, lacerated his face, and shaved his fingertips. Ultimately, he was apprehended and was sent to prison for over twenty years. During his time at Jackson, he was an ideal inmate. He graduated from high school, took college level classes, and started a rose garden on prison grounds. I operated on him in the prison OR (rhinoplasty, face lift, blepharoplasty, and scar revisions.) Fast forward ~2 years. I received a phone call from my Jackson patient, now living in San Francisco. "Hi, Doc, I'm just calling to tell you how well I'm doing. I'm going straight. I have a great job and I'm happily married to my high-school girl friend. She waited for me all those years when I was in prison and Doc, she really needs your help! Would you do some work on her face?" I congratulated him on how well he was doing and referred them to the resident's clinic at UCSF.[17]

## Rotations at the Ann Arbor Veterans Administration Hospital (VA)

The junior resident had some independent responsibility. They ran clinics and scheduled OR cases and received supervision from senior residents and staff. A large majority of the cases were patients with skin cancers and decubitus ulcer, as well as facial shotgun suicide attempts and some hand cases. In addition, a few female patients qualified for reduction mammoplasty, and rarely, we had a face-lift candidate.

## Teaching Conferences
### Tuesday Afternoon Didactic Conference
A wide variety of topics were presented by the resident, faculty, and guest speakers. The schedule was intended to accommodate didactic presentations by individual residents on all the basic science and clinical problems we were encountering in those days. In the beginning, one Tuesday a month was devoted to a review of complicated or preoperative cases that needed staff discussion. We also had visiting Michigan doctors and a number of visiting professors who sometimes operated in the morning with the residents and lectured to the entire staff on their special interest in the afternoon. (See appendix p. 149 for names of some of these visiting professors.) Looking over the yearly reports that are still available, one is impressed by the high caliber of the influences we were exposed to in those days. These included many of the most famous plastic surgeons of their time, who were pioneers in their fields.

### Thursday Morning Conference
As the number of patients grew and we still had limited faculty, more time was needed to discuss the proposed pre-op patients. We moved the patient discussion aspect of the Tuesday conference to Thursday morning, when the entire OR support staff had their weekly meetings and the OR start time was delayed. This gave us time for a more detailed discussion of upcoming cases presented by the residents. Because of conflicting schedules with regard to clinic coverage and the faculty operating in two hospitals, some patients who had not yet been fully evaluated by faculty in the clinic would be presented at the Thursday conference. As a result, it was a very important conference and the residents were put on the spot in terms of their findings and indications for surgery. Frequently, new studies or consultations were recommended by the faculty. The surgical procedure proposed for a patient presented might be modified or, on rare occasions, a nonoperative alternative would be proposed. It became traditional from the outset that *all* faculty made it a point to attend this conference, and the stimulating and open-ended discussions created an excellent and sometimes intimidating teaching experience for both faculty and residents. The students in attendance got a rare and valuable view of informed decision making. The outstanding educational potential of this conference and the support it received from the entire

plastic surgery staff through the years made this an essential event, one that is still on the section's weekly schedule.

We wish to emphasize Bill Grabb's devotion to constantly ensuring improvement in our residents' education. In addition to the series of "ten most wanted" articles (see appendix p. 156) that he brought to everyone's attention, he constantly made suggestions and encouraged (one might say gently demanded) feedback from both residents and faculty. When teaching objectives were modified or expanded, it was always through group input. Any changes made in the conferences themselves were always designed to improve educational opportunities and to keep up to date on new aspects of plastic surgery.

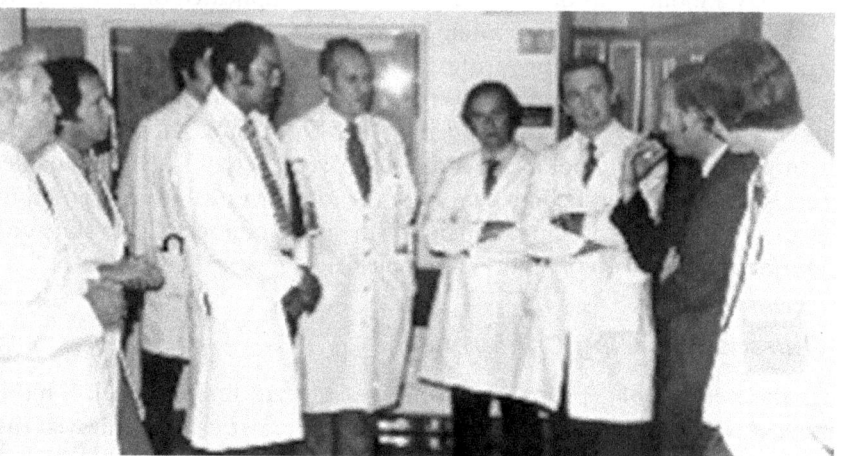

*Photo 45:* Saturday morning patient rounds. From left to right: Drs. Dingman, Novark, Norris, O'Connor, Lawrence, Morris, and Oneal.

## *Saturday Morning Teaching Rounds*

These were "walking rounds" involving all the faculty and residents with bedside visitations to all the patients on the PS service at both SJMH and the university hospital (Photo 45). This ritual was continued for many years. Typically, there would be a long string of more than ten to fifteen of us—faculty, residents, fellows, and students—following Dr. Dingman through a maze of corridors and stairways. Sometimes, we would get distracted and not pay strict attention to where we were going next but would simply follow those in front. In the old university hospital, we would start on the tenth, or sometimes twelfth, floor and wend our way through the private floors and the main wards down to the main floor of the hospital. One morning, the entire group, fortunately all male, followed Dr. Dingman into the men's room. We were all quite embarrassed, but Dr. Dingman did not comment or seem to notice anything unusual.

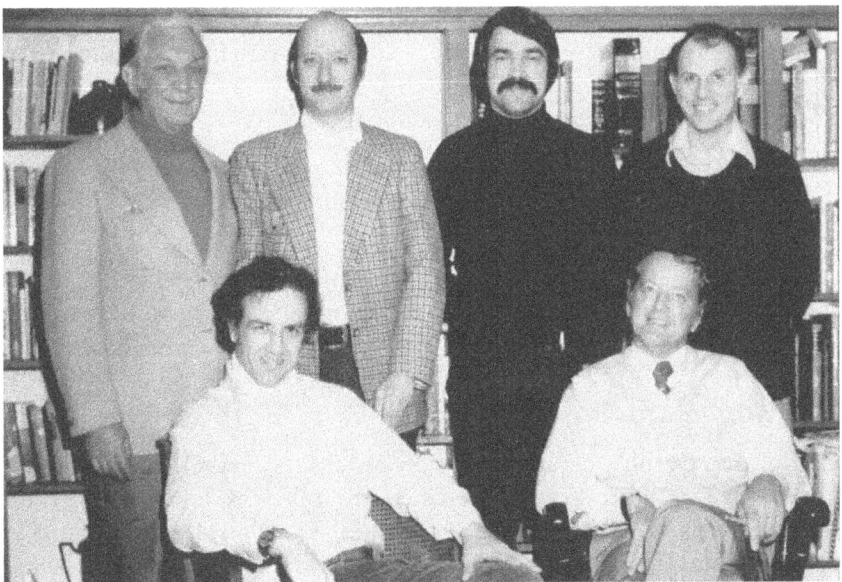

*Photo 46:* Faculty meeting at Dr. Grabb's home: from left to right—front: Drs. Markley and Grabb; rear: Drs. Dingman, Newman, Bucko, and Oneal.

## Weekly Saturday Morning Research Conference

This conference was introduced once Dr. Grabb became section head. The idea was that all the faculty and residents doing research would give a brief report on the progress and new direction of their research projects. He was constantly proposing new ideas and encouraged us all to do the same. He had a wide range of interests that extended beyond traditional plastic surgery that he felt deserved further investigation. The new Sargent laboratory provided an ideal venue for both ongoing and new projects (see chapter six, p. 53, for more details of this lab). He was very receptive to any well-thought-out proposals, and his enthusiasm for research was always in evidence. Dr. Grabb had a nice but firm way of encouraging all of us to be engaged in research. As the number of faculty research projects increased, this conference took on increasing importance. Perhaps once a month all the faculty would meet at Dr. Grabb's home, in his library, and discuss research as well as policies unique to our section (Photo 46).

## Additional Conferences at UMH

*Cleft Lip and Palate: One Saturday Morning a Month*

Attendees included members from plastic surgery, Service of Dentistry, and Department of Speech. The purpose was to discuss the status of current inpatients and also present didactic lectures by staff and invited guests so that all the important aspects of cleft care would be covered in a two-year span.

### Facial Trauma

The conference was held every two months and included members from plastic surgery, dentistry, and otolaryngology (ENT).

### Hand Conference

This was held on the first Saturday of each month and included members of faculty and residents from both plastic surgery and orthopedics.

## Drawing Instruction

During Dr. Grabb's tenure as section head, Dr. Jerry Hodge, the director of medical illustration, offered a course to lead residents through the fundamentals of basic drawing techniques. The course was designed to facilitate and enhance the residents' visual abilities to draw anatomic relationships as well as spatial details of operative techniques. The idea was to improve the residents' artistic appreciations and provide the skill to better illustrate potential procedures, which would improve understanding not only for the residents themselves but also for potential patients. The course was well received, and we all learned that accurate two-dimensional drawings helped to increase our understanding of three-dimensional relationships (Photo 47).

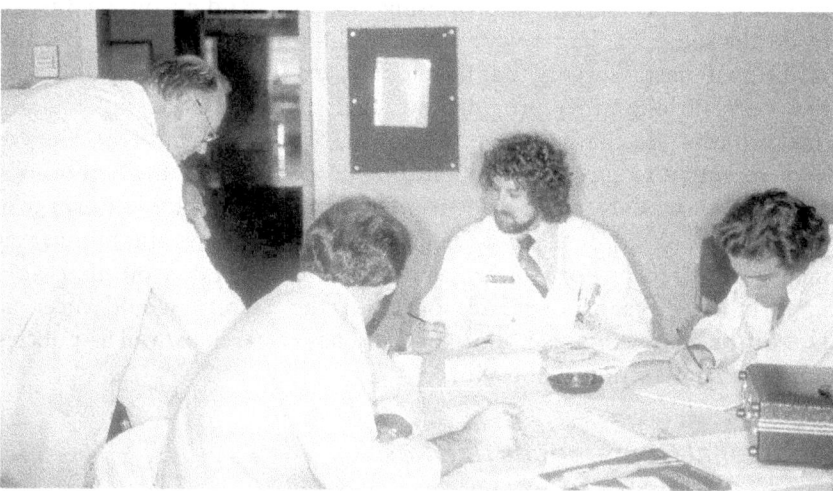

*Photo 47:* Drawing class for residents, directed by Gerald Hodge (standing).

CHAPTER SIX

# Research Activities and the F. Roland Sargent Research Laboratory

Within the academic plastic surgery community, there was general agreement that basic research should be an essential element of any university training program. This was also very high on Dr. Grabb's agenda. Although there were laboratories available at University of Michigan (UM) and the Ann Arbor Veterans Administration (VA) Hospital in which plastic surgical research had been carried out, it was thought that to have a laboratory specifically designated to plastic surgery and independently supported financially would be very desirable for the future growth and success of the program.

The Kresge Research Building, on the corner of Ann Street and Zina Pitcher Street (see Photo 48), housed the medical library as well as research labs that were used by several medical and surgical departments. Dr. Grabb felt strongly that basic laboratory research was of prime importance to the future of plastic surgery and to a successful and well-respected training program. The F. Roland Sargent Research Laboratory, designated for plastic surgery research in Kresge, was donated by Mr. Roland Sargent, a lifelong resident of Saginaw, Michigan, who rose to prominence in the fields of law and road building. He was an admirer of Dr. Grabb's desire to institute a premier research program for faculty and incorporate it into the training of residents and students. The idea of a supported research program was dear to Dr. Grabb's heart, and Mr. Sargent's generosity made this all possible.

An editorial by Dr. Grabb, titled "The Experimental Method," published in *Plastic and Reconstructive Journal* (*PRS*) in 1972,[1] clearly laid out a philosophy for doing research in a university setting. Dr. Grabb stated that he wanted to "light a spark in as many minds as possible on the value of the experimental method" and to "promote a greater

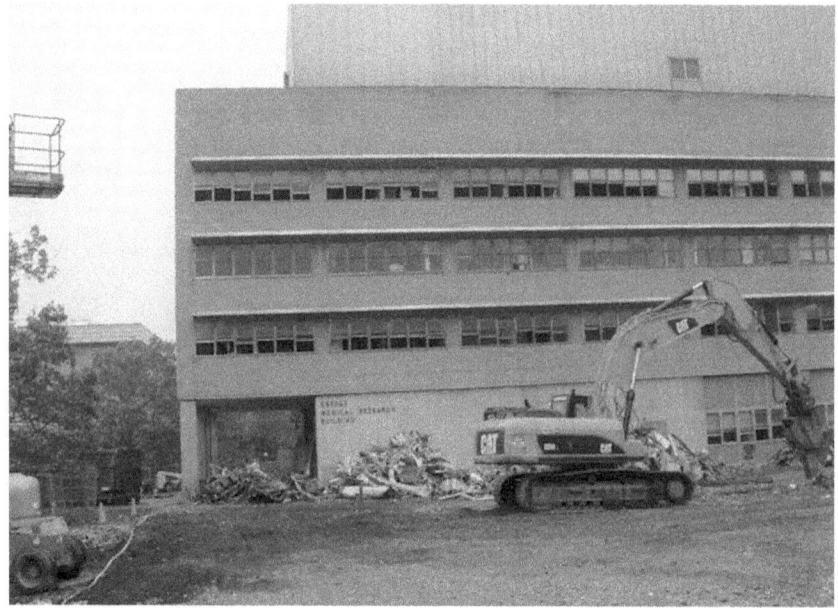

*Photo 48:* Kresge Building in the process of being torn down. Historically, it had been the home of the surgery research labs, medical library, and medical illustration department.

use (of it) in our clinical studies." He further stressed the importance as well as the potential difficulty in designing and carrying out prospective designed studies. He clearly stated the need for careful planning of such studies to achieve one that was random and unbiased. He also emphasized the necessity to "attach validity only to those evaluations that have biostatistical significance" when analyzing results. To facilitate these ideas, he also made a plea for more full-time and adequately funded academic research appointments in university plastic surgery programs. The seeds of the multiuniversity prospective cleft palate study and the full-time faculty and associate research positions in the Section of Plastic Surgery, both of which he eventually achieved to establish, are clearly evident in his editorial.

The laboratory program played an important role in the continued development and growth of the section and quickly became a center for innovative research and resident training, especially in the areas of microsurgery, tissue expansion, the study of flaps, treatment of hemangiomas, and nerve suture techniques. Dr. Grabb was continuously encouraging the faculty and the residents to engage in research projects. He often brought forth lists containing a wide variety of ideas that he was prepared to support. He created an aura of expectation that research was an essential aspect of plastic surgery training

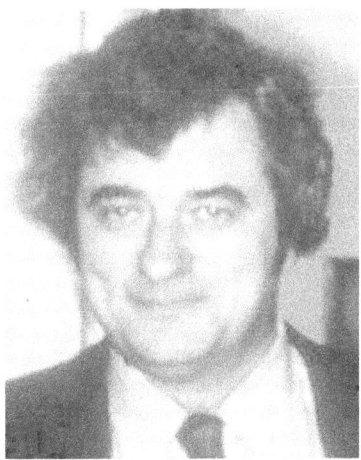

Photo 49: George Cherry, DPhil.

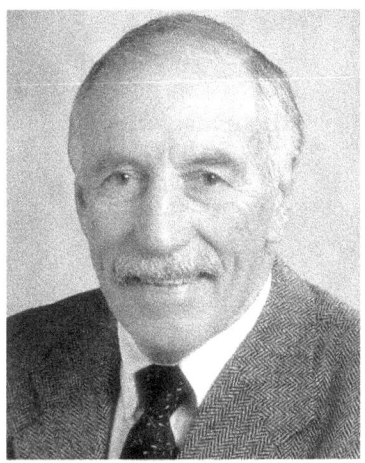

Photo 50: John Faulkner, PhD.

Dr. George Cherry, DPhil, from Oxford, England, was recruited as the director of the laboratory (Photo 49). Later, Dr. Krystyna Pasyk and Dr. Michael Morykwas became important members of the laboratory staff. From the faculty, Dr. Eric Austad and Dr. John Markley were both major contributors with projects in the laboratory from early on. Dr. Austad studied tissue expansion and Dr. Markley studied microvascular surgery and also helped set up a microvascular training program for the residents. We asked both of them to provide, in their own words, the dramatic details of their early projects in the fields of microvascular surgery and skin expansion research.

**Dr. John Markley** described his experience in microvascular research and teaching microvascular techniques:

> In 1977, the first dual binocular operating scope for hand surgery (Zeiss OpMi7) became available, in the newly opened Plastic Surgery lab in the Kresge lab building.
>
> In 1977 John Faulkner [Photo 50] approached Dr. Grabb and asked if we could provide microsurgical help for a series of muscle transplant experiments Dr. Faulkner had in mind. Dr. Grabb asked me to do this. He, Dr. Faulkner, and I met in the North Outpatient PS office to discuss it, and the University of Michigan Department of Physiology/Section of Plastic Surgery muscle physiology collaboration was born.
>
> Dr. Faulkner designed a series of experiments in cats and Rhesus monkeys based on prior work he and others had done. Between 1978 and 1981 I did the surgical procedures with and without

micro-neural anastomoses for these various free and vascular-pedicled muscle transplant experiments on anesthetized cats and monkeys in our Kresge PS lab with our lab operating microscope. The animals were brought to the lab anesthetized, full proper sterile surgical technique was used, and the procedures were done by me with either John Faulkner or Tim White (his post-doc). Subsequent functional, kinetic, and histologic studies and assessments of the results of these operations were done in Dr. Faulkner's lab by his team. This resulted in a series of seven collaborative peer-reviewed journal papers and two book chapters between 1978 and 1989. The findings contributed to both basic science understanding of some physiologic behaviors of transplanted skeletal muscle, and some clinical applicability.

The main findings of this body of work were—

1) Prior work by others had suggested that in order to regenerate any muscle fibers a free (re-vascularized by local vessel ingrowth, not microvascular anastomosis) muscle graft had to be denervated some days or weeks in advance of transplantation. Our work showed this not to be true in cats and monkeys, and subsequently proved out in humans. Non-pre-denervated muscle grafts regenerate and gain functional properties equally well to pre-denervated grafts, thus saving one operation.

2) Motor nerve micro-anastomosis between a muscle grafts' severed motor nerve stump and a recipient area motor nerve improves quality and quantity of regeneration and causes the transplanted muscle fibers to modify to more closely resemble the fiber types and contractile and histochemical properties of muscle normally innervated by the recipient site motor nerve.

3) Temporalis muscle transposed to the face (in place of removed zygomaticus) with vasculature intact but origin and insertion tendons and motor nerve (V) severed and then reinserted with a facial nerve branch micro-anastomosis underwent fiber type changes to more closely resemble facial muscle properties. This even though no muscle fiber degeneration/regeneration took place since the muscle remained perfused at all times. This was analogous to a micro-re-innervated free microvascular muscle flap but without the need for microvascular anastomoses.

4) Regenerated free muscle graft individual fibers develop normal tension for that muscle.

5) Comparing monkey temporalis muscle flaps transposed to the face with continuous perfusion but with severed motor nerve micro-anastomosed to a facial nerve branch, with free muscle

graft with the same micro-neural anastomoses but which had to degenerate and regenerate fibers after vascular ingrowth from adjacent fat and fascia, the free denervated/regenerated grafts developed muscle fiber properties closer to that of facial nerve innervated normal facial muscle. However, this required free grafts of small enough bulk to successfully spontaneously locally re-vascularize.

1978–1983—In addition to using the OpMi scope in the lab for the Faulkner work, the facility was used to teach microvascular technique to the plastic surgery residents. At first, I did this myself, but also trained John Faulkner's lab assistant to do the teaching and she became very proficient and took over the residents' lab anastomotic teaching. In 1978, Paul Izenberg developed a rat hind limb arterial anastomosis patency model with my help in the lab, which he presented to the American College of Surgeons (ACS).[2]

Some of the details of this hind-limb model project were explained by Dr. Izenberg. They included cutting the femoral art and vein and scraping the periosteum, to insure there was no collateral circulation, and leaving the femoral nerve intact to avoid the rat cannibalizing its own leg.[3] Dr. Izenberg won the UM Coller award for this work as well as a prize at the ACS for the best resident's paper in that year. Dr. Hassan Badran, a fellow from Egypt (1978–79), recalled the important role the microvascular lab played in training: "John Markley gave me the first and only lesson in the anastomosis of rat femoral vessels. From there, I took the key to the lab to further train myself based on that single lesson. It helped me to assist in performance of the first thumb replantation in Michigan."[4]

**Dr. Eric Austad**, who was involved from the beginning, recalled the origin and laboratory studies of the development of tissue expansion at UM:

In the summer of 1975, while still a resident in general surgery at Saint Joseph Mercy Hospital in Ann Arbor, I spent a two-month rotation with the plastic surgery service. While working mostly at St. Joe's, I also attended some of the plastic surgery clinics at the university. One of these clinics treated, among a variety of various surgical problems, the patients from Dr. David Schteingart's E&M clinic who had undergone massive weight loss. These losses were often in the 200–400 lb. range, and those patients were often left with festoons of excess skin, which were quite dramatic and disabling. In the same clinic, a subsequent patient might present for reconstruction after a Halsted mastectomy or with a major pressure sore.

This dichotomy, which I came to think of as "the haves and the have-nots," seemed to suggest a new way to approach patients requiring reconstruction after major tissue loss: if skin could expand in surface area to accommodate a major weight gain or, more commonly, to simply grow with an infant into adulthood, a progressively enlarging implant could mimic that process.

Breast implants made of silicone were in wide use at that time, having been developed in the early 1960s, and silicone was the logical material to consider in creating a subcutaneous or submucosal balloon effect. Silicone was generally thought to be nontoxic, inert, and well-tolerated when implanted. Moreover, Dow Corning Medical Products was the major manufacturer of breast implants and a variety of other silicone devices and materials; its primary labs were located only 120 miles north of Ann Arbor, near Midland. I knew that both Dr. Dingman and Dr. Grabb had worked with Dow Corning, and I somehow found the nerve to talk about this concept with each of them individually in the last months of 1975. Even at the time, I knew how audacious this might seem: I wasn't even a plastic surgery resident (yet), and there I was suggesting a way that might lead to a new way of doing things. Dr. Dingman listened patiently to my halting proposal but was not impressed. Dr. Grabb, my only alternative, seemed intrigued, and offered to introduce me to the research group at Dow Corning.

In January of 1976, I drove to Midland and met with six to eight of their science and technical staff. Among them was Silas Braley, arguably Dow Corning's top scientist, though I did not realize his prominence at the time. My main goal was to present the concept of creating new soft tissue with a slowly inflated balloon-like device. A reservoir or valve for filling, attached to the balloon by a tube, was the most obvious design, and I knew from my experience as a neurosurgery resident that implanted fill ports and tubes such as the Rickham Reservoir were currently available. However, the Dow Corning staff did not seem particularly interested, suggesting vaguely that current valve technology was not adequate and that they had already explored similar designs without success. At that point, rather than simply thanking them and returning to Ann Arbor, I described my alternative approach: an osmotically driven implant that would self-inflate with extracellular fluid. I had given this some thought beforehand and was aware of this phenomenon because, as a medical student, I had worked with proteins that were purified by placing dry extracts into sealed, collapsed dialysis tubing and submerging them in saline baths. As if by magic, they would self-inflate as the water component of the saline flowed into them, retaining the large protein molecules but washing away impurities in the process. The need for valves and tubing could be eliminated, as well as repeated incremental inflations and the risk of at least some human error. This was more interesting to the Dow Corning staff, and to me.

At the time of my visit to Dow Corning, I was not aware that a plastic surgery resident at Georgetown, Chedomir Radovan, MD, was already developing what would become known as the Radovan Expander. In fact, his first expander was placed at Georgetown on January 26, 1976, only a few weeks after my Dow Corning visit. While my concept of tissue expansion came from my exposure to massive weight-loss patients, I learned later, in talking with him, that Radovan conceived his version by observing his wife's pregnant abdomen a year earlier. In fact, neither of us was aware that the concept of "tissue expansion" had actually been developed, and the phrase coined, by a New York plastic surgeon, Charles G. Neumann. A few years ago, I had talked with one of Dr. Neumann's former residents at Bellevue, Dr. James Lawson, who recalled fabricating some of those first expanders by gluing (somehow) condoms to the tubing of Foley catheters in the mid-1950s. In any case, Neumann's pioneering work with tissue expansion was presented to the ASPRS (that was the society's name then) and published in 1958, but it was met with little interest and was apparently forgotten by most of his colleagues. Neither Radovan nor I was aware of Neumann's work until the mid-1980s.

Unaware of Radovan's work and wishing to develop a silicone self-inflating expander, I knew that both the permeability characteristics of silicone and its optimal contents were key features. I assumed that Dow Corning, with its already vast experience with a variety of silicone applications, could tell me how their medical-grade product behaved as a semi-permeable membrane. In fact, at that time they had no idea, or at least any information they believed they could share. They did indicate, however, that sodium chloride, plain table salt, was known to be relatively inhibited from crossing a silicone barrier. As a major component of extracellular fluid and a relatively nontoxic material, this salt seemed a logical candidate to provide an osmotic driving force from inside a silicone implant shell. Moreover, the molecular weight of its component ions, sodium and chloride, were both low. This meant that on a weight-for-weight basis, it would be more osmotically efficient than larger molecules such as proteins. With all of that in mind, Dow Corning agreed to provide testicular-sized implant shells sealed and containing varying selected weights of sodium chloride. At that point, we had no idea whether, or at what rate, these implants might inflate when placed in saline baths. When we found that these first implants invariably floated to the surface, making their surface area in contact with the saline baths inconsistent, we modified the bath containers to allow the implants to be suspended beneath the surface by tethers of thin monofilament line. Subsequently, these baths resembled miniatures of the harbors of World War II, which had been mined with spherical explosives. In retrospect, that might have provided a note of caution.

The permeability studies continued through late 1976 and most of 1977, but we learned early that the basic concept appeared good. Silicone shells of the usual medical-grade thickness did indeed "draw in" water from a saline bath at a predictable rate, but that rate was lower than we hoped. Unless enough sodium chloride was added to them to maintain a saturated solution throughout inflation, rates to full inflation required months rather than weeks. These data were all contained as part of our first presentation of our experience at the annual meeting of the ASPRS in Toronto in 1979, defining for the first time the permeability coefficient of medical grade silicone to water. At that time, I was working in the F. Roland Sargent Laboratory of the Section of Plastic Surgery with Dr. Cherry, and undergraduate students Greg Rose and Steve Thomas. All three remained highly involved with this and subsequent work involving self-inflating expanders, and Krystyna Pasyk, MD, joined us when histological studies became more pertinent in late 1977. With this team of four colleagues, we felt ready to begin animal experiments with guinea pigs in the fall of 1977.

As regards tissue expansion, my work in my resident years 1977–80 was primarily focused on the basic research noted previously, and Bill Grabb continued to be a major supporter and guide. Work with the self-inflating expander continued, and in 1979, it was awarded first prize in the Clinical Category of the annual meeting of the ASPRS research competition. My paper, though primarily limited to guinea pig studies, argued strongly for the basic safety of tissue expansion, finding no evidence of ominous mitotic changes, vascular disruption, nerve damage, or changes in hair distribution. We could not yet identify the origin of this expanded tissue, as we could not discern an increase in mitosis with our limited histological techniques, but I believe that this work was critical for the ongoing use of the technique. No one had previously studied any of the actual histology and tissue changes of expansion. At this same meeting, Radovan presented for the first time his experience with impressive reconstructions using expansion (as noted, his previous two presentations were "poster sessions," with limited exposure). With good support for the basic safety and efficacy of tissue expansion, the technique rapidly became mainstream.

While tissue expansion was becoming a common technique worldwide, basic questions remained regarding the quality of the tissue it generated. It seemed to work, but how, and why? In 1982 Drs. Krystyna Pasyk [see Group Photo 1982], Ken McClatchey [Photo 51], and I reported more detail in P&RS on the basic histology of expansion, emphasizing its basic safety, but issues remained regarding the reliability of expanded flaps. Specifically, was vascularity sufficient to support major flaps? At that point in time, flap delay was the only technique known to increase survival, based primarily on the work of Stuart Milton at Oxford. George Cherry was a colleague of Milton at Oxford, and we were fortunate to have him subsequently at Michigan. Dr. Cherry adapted Milton's protocols using expanded flaps in adult pigs (no casual feat), and Drs. Cherry, Rod Rohrich, and I were the first to report that expansion actually results in increased flap survival and vascularity, comparable to the delay phenomenon. This finding has persisted and has been replicated by others. It remains a key feature of expansion and has been relied upon routinely in difficult surgical situations.

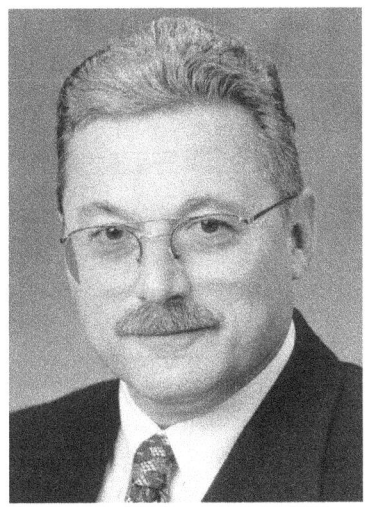

Photo 51: Ken McClatchey, DDS, MD.

As surgeons were gaining and reporting new and innovative clinical work with expansion throughout the 1980s, and Michigan was well-represented among them, we also continued to wrestle with the basic problem of silicone permeability. We found in early studies that a puncture or leak of a salt-containing implant at the time of placement was not problematic: the salt inside would simply dissolve and leak slowly into the extracellular space, causing no harm. However, we did not realize that this was not the worst-case situation. In fact, tissue loss did occur when an implant containing the high volume of salt needed for more-rapid inflation was purposely ruptured near full inflation. It appeared that the sudden burst of saturated saline solution from the implant was not tolerated in the guinea pig model we used: although no animals died, some necrosis occurred and we clearly needed to modify the model if it was to be widely used. The tissue loss was no worse than that seen with partial loss of a conventional flap, but these implants represented a product liability situation not associated with flaps. We tried thinner silicone shells, but those proved unreliable. We tried silicone shells containing sodium chloride crystals, but they did not significantly increase inflation characteristics. We tried silicone shells with "windows" of more permeable material, without benefit. We even tried ion sputtering, working with the university engineers, without success. The basic problem with the self-inflating implant remained technical: silicone, in its usual medical-grade configuration or the modifications we tried, was simply not permeable enough to water. I continued to believe that the right material(s) were "out there somewhere," but by the late 1980s, the basic safety of silicone as an implantable material was being questioned. As virtually all of the implant manufacturers I worked with left the field and/or closed, our work stopped, and did not resume.

As my last and, I believe, most significant contribution to tissue expansion research, I had been vitally interested in the actual origin of expanded tissue since my earliest work with the technique. It was clear that tissue could be expanded, sometimes to an unbelievable extent, but where did it all come from? The only work that was pertinent to this question was that in our previously noted first paper, which addressed the basic safety of expansion but could not demonstrate an increase in mitotic activity using standard H&E stains. An alternative to actual increased mitosis was the theory that "creep" was the active mechanism: simple stretching. I didn't believe this was the only process at work, particularly in view of the increased vascularity and flap strength we had previously reported. With the help of Krystyna Pasyk and Steve Thomas, we eventually studied mitotic rates of expanding guinea pig skin using a more-sensitive isotopic technique. Tritiated thymadine was used to label cells undergoing mitosis and we clearly showed in guinea pigs that mitosis was significantly increased after each incremental inflation of a Radovan-type expander. Moreover, mitotic activity decreased from baseline when implant volume was decreased, indicating an exquisite interplay between growth requirements and cell responses. Our 1986 paper in P&RS was titled "Tissue Expansion: Dividend or Loan?" I believe that we answered that now-rhetorical question, and answered it first. To my knowledge, its conclusions have never been contradicted."[5]

## Other Important Laboratory Projects

### Lab Projects Directed at the Study of Skin Flaps

Dr. Grabb and a variety of associates, including Dr. Cherry, Dr. Manders, and Richard Faller, worked on several projects regarding skin flaps from 1978 to 1980. (Dr. Faller was a premed student who was a loyal worker in several laboratory projects. He is a good example of the highly dedicated kind of people, who are so essential to any successful lab program.) Some of the aspects studied were the effect of tourniquet ischemia, effects of gravity, tissue fibrinolytic activity, and isopurine and microcirculatory changes after flap elevation.

Dr. Ron Wexler, who completed residency in 1972, went back to Jerusalem and Hadassah Hospital, where he became chief of plastic surgery. During the summer of 1980, at Dr. Grabb's invitation, he spent a three-month sabbatical working in the Sargent laboratory. He completed a number of projects with various collaborators, for example, a study with Neil Ford Jones (resident in 1980) to help define pressure bursa limits that "allows minimal removal of adjacent normal tissue,"[6] a description of a visual method to measure size and shape of skin flaps in pigs,[7] and a study to evaluate better survival in small skin flaps. The study showed that the flap should be broadened immediately adjacent to its short narrow base, giving it a tree foliage pattern; thus, an arbor (shaped) flap not a rectangular one[8] and another explaining the concept of "perfusion takeover."[9] Ron was very enthusiastic about this research, and he specifically and especially gives credit to Dr. George Cherry and Mr. Richard Faller. He also spoke admiringly of James Crudup and the rest of the excellent animal care staff and the Department of Medical Photography.[10]

Another project that was supported by Dr. Grabb took place in 1973–74 and was reported by Dr. James Norris: "Larry Wisenthall, a fourth-year medical student, and I (then a senior resident) were investigating methods to increase skin flap survival. I felt that nicotine was a definite factor in the survival of flaps and we set out to study this problem. Dr. Grabb helped secure the lab facilities for us and I bought the rabbits. Dr. Grabb wanted us to present our work at the Educational Foundation annual conference, but Larry and I felt that we needed to do more. Unfortunately, I left and Larry had to focus on his internship so that ended the project."[11]

Attempting to find a fluorescent chemical to delineate adequate blood supply that did not turn patients yellow as the highly effective fluorescein did (see p. 86 under "Skin Flaps" section for information about the successful use of fluorescein) led to the discovery of esculin, the story of which is described in Lauralee's own words:

> Dr. Grabb wanted every resident to participate in RESEARCH, indicating that this activity was not voluntary. One afternoon after once again typing research reminders to all residents, it struck me that research was something I could do. So I went to Dr. Grabb and announced that I would go home that night and come back the next

morning with an answer he had been seeking. I would find a clear, fluorescent, injectable material to replace Sodium Fluorescein used in flap surgery (to determine flap viability after the flap had been raised). The new drug would have the advantage of not turning the patient yellow. That evening I was reading a garden book and found the answer. I learned that the bark of Horse Chestnut trees (*Aesculus rubicunda*) had properties (esculin) that fluoresced with a clear, white light. I closed the book and felt I found what I wanted. The next day, I phoned Richard Faller in our lab and asked him to look in a catalog to see if esculin was available. He did, and it was a $5.00 for five grams. Then I asked Dr. Grabb to authorize this expense so esculin could be tested [for safety and efficacy] and then used on our lab animals. Esculin did work on flaps in various animals and Richard's subsequent photographs documented the extent of blood circulation in the raised flaps. Ultimately this work led to a US patent in my name. Dr. Eric Austad knew the ropes of getting a patent and became my sine qua non. Later, Dr. Lou Argenta and Dr. Dingman arranged a meeting for a group from Dow Corning to come to Ann Arbor to hear about esculin, including a demonstration, and perhaps fund additional studies. Dow showed an interest but did not want to pursue it as it was not yet tested on humans. To date, the patent remains dormant but I continue to be a proud patent holder.[12]

## *Nerve Suturing Techniques in Monkeys*

In this study, Dr. Grabb collaborated with members of the UM School of Engineering and Department of Physical Medicine in the UM Medical School.[13] Three techniques of nerve suture repair of transected ulnar nerves in monkeys were evaluated. The results demonstrated that direct fascicular suturing improved results over simple epineural suturing. The other significant finding was that defining specific motor and sensory fascicles electrically did not improve the results over careful lining up of the fascicles in relation to their size and position.

Drs. Bucko and Grabb reported a study on the effect of D-pennicillamine-induced lathyrism on nerve regeneration in monkeys.[14] Dr. Bucko reported that "while at Utah in General Surgery residency, he started a project to minimize scarring around primate autographs. He had an NIH training grant in immunology. He continued this work when he came to Ann Arbor and with Dr. Grabb's help got a grant and procured a colony of spider monkeys to work with. He was using (beta-aminoproprionitrile fumarate), BAPN, which was suggested by work done by Krizek and Robson at Yale." He also stated that they had a lot of trouble keeping the monkeys alive under the influence of the drug treatment and he felt the results on nerve regeneration were inconclusive.[15] One interesting anecdote is, as L3 recalls to the best of her memory, getting a call from the director at the primate lab at the VA hospital where Dennis had his monkeys. The monkeys had apparently removed the postsurgical dressing and gotten out of their cages, and it was quite an adventure getting them back in.[16]

CHAPTER SEVEN

# Clinical Research, Clinical Procedures, New Techniques—1946–86

After discussion among the authors, editors, and contributors to this book, it was decided to describe as succinctly as possible the clinical activities of Drs. Dingman (ROD) and Grabb (WCG) leading up to 1964. Beyond that point, we decided to provide a sampling of the expanding clinical activities by categories rather than solely in historical order. In addition, we asked our colleagues Drs. Markley and Austad, as well as Dr. Hack Newman, to provide their personal recollections of three important clinical areas that contributed to define this highly innovative and transformative era of plastic surgery history: replantation and free tissue transfer, clinical use of expansion, and the development of craniofacial surgery at the University of Michigan (UM).

### Early Work of Dr. Dingman and Dr. Grabb

Prior to his plastic surgery training with Dr. Ferris Smith that was completed in 1946, Dr. Dingman's curriculum vitae (CV) indicated his clinical activity was mostly limited to oral surgery conditions and concerns. One exception was an article in 1939 in the *Archives of Otolaryngology* about periocular sinuses. The other published subjects include management of facial fractures, osteomyelitis and tumors of the jaws, abnormalities of the temporomandibular joint (TMJ), and orthognathic surgery. However, beginning in 1948 and up until Dr. Grabb joined him in 1961, Dr. Dingman's emphasis shifted to subjects more of an interest to plastic surgeons. In 1948, he published an article on surgical correction of developmental deformities of the mandible in the second volume of *the Plastic and Reconstructive Surgery (PRS) journal*.[1] This was followed by articles on such varied subjects as cleft lip,[2] *iliac* bone grafts,[3] malunion of facial fractures,[4] Z-plasty,[5] radiated costal cartilage,[6] ostectomy of the mandible in cleft lip and cleft palate patients,[7] and rhinoplasty caused by defects of the septum.[8] In 1961, when Dr. Grabb was a resident and coauthor, two articles were published, one on lymphangioma of the tongue[9] and the other on human rib cartilage grafts preserved by irradiation.

The latter article turned out to be an important contribution to facial reconstruction. The following is quoted from the introduction to the 1961 *PRS* article by Dingman and Grabb[10]: "Preserved costal cartilage homografts have proven to be of value in restoring contour defects of the supporting structures of the face. The cartilage can be sterilized and preserved indefinitely. It can be easily sculptured at the operating table and after implantation it is well tolerated by the body tissue." Dr. Dingman quoted an earlier article from 1956,[11] where he and two others reported the use of irradiation to sterilize canine costal cartilage, and it was subsequently determined that sterilization of human costal cartilage could be accomplished by rapid (fifteen hours) cobalt 69 gamma irradiation using 3,000,000 rep. This was carried out in the Ford Nuclear Reactor in the Phoenix Memorial Laboratory at the UM.

The cartilage was obtained at autopsy, ideally from young adults, and was refrigerated and stored until it could be prepared by a resident assigned to this project. The cartilage was stripped of soft tissues and the perichondrium was preserved. It was then cut into lengths to fit into a glass canning jar filled with saline and tightly sealed. After sterilization by the irradiation, the cartilage is ready for use the next day or can be stored indefinitely. The article reported that twenty-eight of thirty human patients receiving these grafts for chin augmentation, orbital floor defects, and dorsum of the nose showed no clinical evidence of absorption in seven months to 3½ years postoperatively. (The two that absorbed were used for external ear reconstruction where autologous cartilage is essential for success.) This knowledge of the successful utilization of homograft cartilage was essential in our reconstructive efforts as there were few other materials available or more dependable for many years after this report. We all kept a few of these jars containing the irradiated cartilage close at hand in the operating room (OR) suite for many years. Illustrative of Dr. Dingman's intellectual generosity is the statement in the summary in the 1961 article that the arrangements for the resources of the Phoenix lab at the UM would be available for others interested in adopting this technique.[12] Dr. Wexler sent his recollection about the cartilage collection (which has undergone some minor editing):

> Twice a month we went to the morgue, opened chests, cutting the out cartilaginous part of the ribs [cutting ribs in to 4 cm lengths], then put them into saline-filled transparent glass jars. They were taken to the atomic reactor on North Campus, irradiated with 3 million rads

and the jars became brown. We kept the jars on the shelves ready to be used as filling material—similar to the silicones today. This was excellent, curvable, infection resistant material. One evening, in the winter, I took a bar [of cartilage] to be used at Jackson prison. I left it in my car. Next morning I found a block of ice in the car surrounded with broken glass. What happened to the cartilage? I do not recall exactly. Why might it have been taken and what to be used for?[13]

Paul Izenberg recalled six years later that the cadaver cartilage was still being collected: "I remember being called into the section office by Lauralee and being told 'it's time' knowing that the task of harvesting cartilage for processing was upon us. So a couple of us (usually junior residents) hiked over the cadaver lab to process the specimens."[14] Paul suggests that this denatured homograft material was, in a way, a forerunner of acellular dermal matrix, now one of the most often used homografts in plastic surgery.[15]

In further review of Dr. Dingman's CV, it was noted that starting around the time in 1952 when he turned down the chairmanship of oral surgery at the dental school and aligned himself with the surgery department at the medical school, he had published a series of articles during the subsequent ten years, either collaborating with someone from another specialty in the medical center or on a subject only peripherally related to plastic surgery but published in one of the other specialty journals. Examples include an article about Z-plasty to the urethral meatus, published with Dr. Reed Nesbit who was chairman of the urology department; an article about cheilitis glandularis with reconstruction of the upper lip, with Dr. Arthur "Whitey" Curtis who was head of the dermatology department; and an article about semi-open burn management, with Dr. Irving Feller, a member of the general surgery section and on his way to becoming a burn specialist who was responsible for setting up the Burn Unit at UM. Examples of the second category include an article about necrobiosis lipoidica diabeticorum published in *AMA Archives of Dermatology and Syphilology* 1951,[16] one regarding a malunion of the zygoma in the *Transactions of the American Academy of Ophthalmology*,[17] and another about a burn scar contracture of the neck in the *Surgery Clinics of North America*. While noting the subjects and coauthors of these various publications, it occurred to me that perhaps during those ten or so years, Dr. Dingman was making a concerted effort to reach out and show the applicability of basic plastic surgery principles in the management of a wide variety of medical and surgical problems. He was also trying to heighten awareness of the value of having plastic surgery as a readily available consulting service within a major medical center. Perhaps just as important were his efforts toward building rapport among the medical staff to gain support for the ultimate formation of a plastic surgery section in the medical center within the Department of Surgery.

Subsequently, the range of continuing and varied interests, as shown in his list of publications, continued to expand rapidly. Some of the subjects included management of tumors, wound healing, and Z-plasty. A particular interest involved facial injuries associated with auto accidents. This led to a series of articles from 1960 to 1968, published together with Dr. Grabb and Dr. Donald Huelke, a professor in the anatomy department and a research scientist at the UM Transportation Research Institute. The subjects included facial injuries due to windshield impacts injuries and deaths from windshield and instrument panel impacts. One of the most significant findings, published in 1968, concerned the decrease in frequency and severity of facial lacerations after introduction of the new automobile windshield design.[18] This new design almost single-handedly eradicated the frequent and extensive facial lacerations (one to three patients a week seen in our emergency rooms) that resulted from the vehicle's occupant's head penetrating the older design windshields in front-end collisions (no seat belts in those days).

Along the way, new instruments were introduced. The first was a bone and cartilage grasping forceps in 1954[19] that became widely used. The next was a newly designed plastic surgery dressing cart for use in hospitals and modifiable for use in other specialties. The details of the design were published in 1957 with coauthors Dr. Paul Natvig, who was still a plastic surgery resident, and Jim Winkler, who was then a resident in general surgery at Saint Joseph Mercy Hospital (SJMH).[20] In 1965, with Dr. Grabb as coauthor, Dr. Dingman introduced the now universally used Dingman mouth gag for cleft palate repair in 1962 (discussed, with photo, on pp. 99–100).[21] He also developed the double-ended Dingman periosteal elevator, the Dingman ear abrader (described under the discussion of otoplasty, p. 107), and the transaxillary augmentation mammoplasty dissector (described in the section on augmentation mammoplasty, p. 90).

It is difficult to summarize the enormous clinical output of the next several years. Dr. Dingman's interest in innovations and clinical problems encompassed a wide range of subjects in addition to those already mentioned: facial reconstruction; face, brow, and eyelid surgery; rhinoplasty; otoplasty; scalp and lip reconstruction; cleft lip repair; other developmental abnormalities; chest wall reconstruction; treatment of multiple types of benign and malignant lesions; and TMJ surgery.

In 1964, there was an important article on TMJ reconstruction with metatarsal grafts by Dr. Dingman with Dr. Grabb as coauthor.[22]

The article reported and described the technique Dr. Dingman developed for treating a twenty-nine-year-old female to correct the deformity resulting from a previous operation, ten years earlier, when a surgeon had removed her bilateral mandibular condyles as a radical method to treat intractable TMJ symptoms. On presentation, she had a severe open bite with only her molar teeth in occlusion. Restoration of the condyles was accomplished by using the heads of the bilateral fifth metatarsal bones as fresh autogenous grafts. The patient was followed for seventeen months, and x-rays showed transplanted bone to be intact, and normal occlusion and mandibular function restored, with markedly improved speech. She had no complaints with her feet and was wearing only a slightly narrower shoe than before. The authors drew the conclusion that half-joint transplants do not undergo the destructive changes of bone and cartilage that occur in whole joint transplants. This was a very significant finding. Interestingly, several months later, the patient had an irradiated costal cartilage graft to correct her retruding chin deformity. A 1975 article (referenced and discussed in p. 114) reported an additional eight more cases using metatarsal grafts in a variety of deformities of the TMJ, all with satisfactory results.

There were several articles published and many coauthored with Dr. Grabb on various aspects of both acute traumatic and secondary deformities of facial bones. Of course, the highpoint of the published work on that subject was Drs. Dingman and Natvig's book titled *Surgery of Facial Fractures*, published in 1964 (Photo 52). It became the "bible" for the treatment of facial fractures (referenced and discussed in p. 112). Dr. Dingman always encouraged and invited both his colleagues and residents to join him in these many projects that resulted in publications. That continued well beyond his retirement as section head.

In those early years, in addition to Dr. Grabb and myself, there were faculty members from many disciplines as coauthors with Dr. Dingman. These included Dr. Harlan Bloomer, director of the speech clinic; Dr. Donald Huelke; Gerald Hodge, head of medical

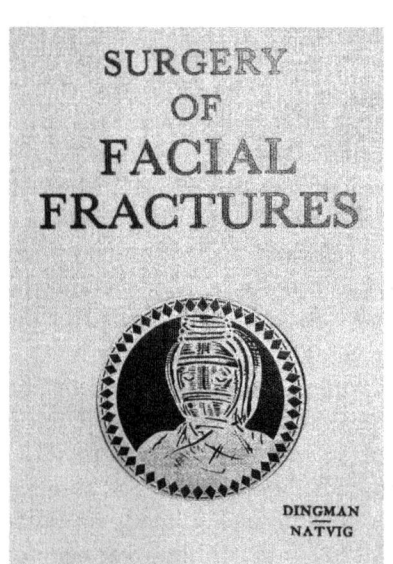

Photo 52: Cover of the book, Surgery of Facial Fractures.

illustration; and Dr. Robert Ponitz, DDS, an orthodontist in private practice who worked closely with all of us in our orthognathic cases as well as consulting in the SJMH Cleft Palate Clinic. The list also includes Krystyna Pasyk, PhD, who was an active participant for many years in the Sargent laboratory, and Dr. Gary Sandall, a pediatric ophthalmologist. Examples from the resident/fellow group of coauthors through these years and beyond include James Winkler; Jim Bennett; Bob Knode; Ralph Seaton; John Markley, who was a student at the time; Eric Constant; Don Davis; Grant Fairbanks; Ron Wexler; Joe Agris; Bob Wilensky; Isaac Peled; Paul Izenberg; Paul Dempsey; Paul Natvig; Bob Gilman; and Malcolm Marks.

When Dr. Grabb completed his residency, he joined Dr. Dingman in practice at SJMH. From the very beginning, he brought innumerable ideas and much energy to the academic side of the residency training program. One example is the clinical study of the anatomy of the mandibular ramus of the seventh nerve published together with Dr. Dingman in 1962.[23] One hundred human facial halves were dissected with cooperation from Dr. Russell Woodburn, head of the Department of Anatomy. Dr. Woodburn was a wonderful and inspiring teacher and friend to all surgeons who were interested in the details of anatomy. This study, carried out on embalmed cadavers, defined that the position of the mandibular ramus, *anterior* to the facial artery, was always above the lower border of the mandible. At the posterior, the branch or branches were often below the mandibular border, and this was a warning to the surgeon approaching this area to undertake an open reduction of the mandible. This study was well received and referred to often in the OR.

Breaking new ground, five years later, Dr. Grabb published an important study that described and clarified the characteristics of the first and second branchial arch syndrome.[24] This syndrome was defined as a constellation of abnormalities resulting in a spectrum of facial malformations that blend with one another and have no bold or clear lines of delineation. The paper was based on a study of 102 patients who were identified by birth records at SJMH and who agreed to return for clinical evaluation. This was a pioneering study and very well regarded at the time. It was an important step leading to a new and clearer idea of a "sequence," which defines the spectrum of anomalies found within types of congenital facial deformities.

As mentioned in detail under his tenure as section head and so beautifully stated in Dr. Dingman's eulogy, Bill Grabb was a prolific researcher, writer, and teacher in addition to being an inspirational and highly respected leader.

## Categories of Clinical Activities
### *Hand Surgery*

Up to 1974, Bill Grabb, John Tipton (until 1969), and I managed the majority of soft tissue injuries of the hand and forearm at SJMH. Most of the hand trauma in that period at the UM was taken care of on the orthopedic service unless directly referred to plastic surgery. A lot of upper extremity tendon and nerve injuries, as well as some quite serious soft tissue trauma and burns, came under our care, which nicely augmented the experience our residents were having on the Detroit Hand Service rotation. In 1967, ROD, WCG, and I published in the Michigan State medical journal, an update on current use of flexor tendon grafts.[25] Later, because of the common postgraft tendon adhesion that occurred in the more complex injuries and limited tendon excursion, we began to use, in badly traumatized injuries, the "Hunter silicone rod" technique. These rods were placed into the palm and fingers to stimulate a new tendon sheath with less chance of forming adhesions after the tendon graft was placed in a secondary procedure.

At SJMH, we usually collaborated with orthopedic consultants when there were associated bony injuries. They were happy to share in the tendon repair work after there was an accidental medial nerve stripping on their service in an attempt to procure a palmaris longus graft. One of the cases I did early in my practice illustrated the principle of sharing part of a nonfunctional digit to restore function in an essential digit. The patient had a partial amputation of his dominant thumb just distal to the M-P joint and of his adjacent index finger through the mid-proximal phalanx. This injury resulted in a nonfunctional, too-short thumb and a nonuseful index finger stump that was in the way. A neurovascular transfer of the residual index finger phalanx to lengthen the residual thumb and a ray amputation of the second metacarpal restored sensate thumb function for pinch and grasp and eliminated the in-the-way index digit. That case made me realize I had made the right choice in becoming a plastic surgeon.

John Markley provided his recollections of the hand program at the UM from 1974 to 1984:

> I was interviewed by Dean Louis in May 1974 as part of the process of my appointment to start in July 1974, at which time I suggested forming a combined Plastic Surgery-Orthopedic Surgery hand service. He was not at all interested, and we agreed to co-exist amicably and compete. At that time orthopedics did not have any microsurgical capability.
>
> When I started in 1974, I was named director of the Plastic Surgery Hand Service, and started a one-afternoon-a-week hand

clinic, staffed by me, with one resident (sometimes two, a junior and a senior), and Loraine Smith, one of our nursing aides [Photo 53]. This started out slowly but it gradually built, and had a big boost with the first digital replant I did in 1976 (first in Michigan). Numerous replant cases followed. In addition, I did the first two microsurgical free toe-to-hand transfers in 1978 and 1979 with the residents at that time. However, beyond the microsurgery, the overall hand experience grew nicely. I lobbied and educated other specialties, for example, pediatrics, neurology, rheumatology, emergency medicine, and so on, and cases came in from all those and continued until I left in July 1983. Between then and 1984, I continued to see problem hand cases once a month in the UM Hand Clinic on a consultant basis for cases selected by Dr. Tom Stevenson.

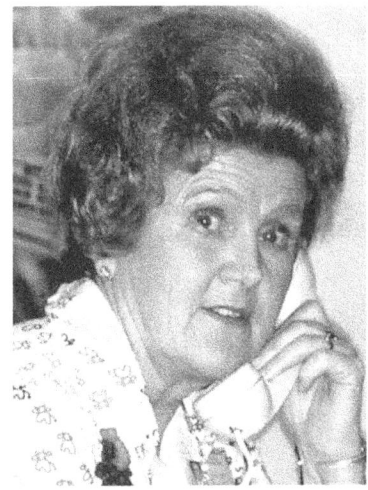

*Photo 53:* Loraine Smith, LPN, a devoted and highly skilled assistant and clinic nurse.

I started the annual hand/forearm gross anatomy dissection series, three 1.5 hour dissections each fall in 1980 and continued that every year [until I retired in 2007].[26]

This is another excellent example of the great teaching value created by the availability of fresh cadaver anatomy specimens. (There is now a videotape of one of his dissections in the residents' online teaching library.)

Markley continued,

> The part of the timeline that I cannot fully recall, nor do I have any records to help, is this. When I started in 1974, the residents were still going to Detroit for additional hand experience. That did not stop until I had been doing the hand clinic for a while (probably about 1982). In addition, at some point in the 1976–1978 time frame, I started teaching the residents micro-neurovascular suture technique using rats in the Kresge [Sargent] lab. However, somewhere in that time I advised sending the residents to Louisville for Bob Acland's week-long microsurgical courses and that was done, I think until 1983–84.

Markley continued, discussing hand joint replacement with silicone implants:

> The metacarpal-phalangeal (MPJ) implants and the interphalangeal joint (IPJ) implants are identical, just different sizes. I'm not sure when I first used the smaller ones in IPJs but likely within a couple years after 1976. The thing is, the indications for use in metacarpal and interphalangeal joints are all different somewhat, and less common in the IPJs than in MPJs. In the MPJs, the indication is nearly always rheumatoid, occasionally trauma or degenerative. They are rarely indicated in the DIJs where usually fusion is better. They work very well in individual PIJs with post-traumatic or osteoarthritis, under some circumstances, and I used them there much more than in DIJs but less frequently than MPJs. Use in IPJs is more technically demanding to get a good result since the silastic does bend laterally as well as dorso-volar, which is not a problem in MPJs but requires careful attention to ligamentous lateral stability in IPJs.[27]

One contribution John did not mention was the excellent *PRS* article he published in 1977 describing digital neurovascular island flaps and the discussion of two-point discrimination achieved.[28] In addition, I am a personal recipient of John Markley's skill by virtue of an indicis proprius tendon transfer to repair a spontaneous ruptured extensor pollicis longus on my dominant hand in 1975 that to this day is functioning perfectly.

## *Treatment of Skin Cancers*

In 1969, in a report in the UM medical journal from members of the Section of Plastic Surgery, the authors presented a statistical evaluation of treatment of basal cell and squamous cell carcinoma in 653 UM patients treated through 1961, thus allowing a five-year follow-up period.[29] Of great significance was the opportunity to use the university's IBM 7090 computer, which allowed the analysis of the effect of a large number of factors on the cure rates and specifically the variables and treatments that were related to recurrences. Following are two of the most significant conclusions: significance of the specific type of treatment-affected cure rates was at the .05 confidence level and electrodessication and curettage was the most effective treatment and radiation therapy the least in producing cure rates. Location of tumors most likely to recur included lateral nose, internal nares, and external auditory canal. Ulceration-invasive growth pattern and multicentric appearance were also prominent factors for recurrence. The final comments of the authors included, "It is likely that methods of treating skin cancers have improved since 1961, when our present study ended." It was thought that more effective treatment had been brought about by the following factors: (1) the use of Mohs's chemosurgical method (Dr. Mohs reported a 0.9 percent recurrence rate in four thousand cases using his technique in a personal communication to the lead author), (2) all radiation therapy was now being given in a new unit by highly improved techniques, (3) most surgical treatments for skin cancers were now handled in the Section of Plastic Surgery. There were three important aspects of this study: an advanced computer was used for analysis; authorship included a medical student (Jesselson) and a plastic surgery resident (Dr. Seaton), an important factor in their education; and results of the study positively affected the subsequent management of these types of lesions. It was clear that complete excision of the lesion at the time of primary operation was essential to lowering the recurrence rate. To achieve this would require close collaboration with a clinical pathologist at the time of primary excision. In addition, the use of the Mohs technique should be strongly considered for specific difficult lesions.

We all saw patients with parts of their faces eaten away as a result of inadequately treated basal cell cancers. Thus, we were always looking for the most effective way of treating these lesions primarily. Our first line of action was a close collaboration at the time of initial excision with our pathologists at SJMH. We would do the initial excision with an adequate visual margin. Before completely removing the lesion, we would mark the specimen with a suture at one edge for orientation. Then we would take the specimen over to the pathology department and, together with the pathologist, decide the technique that would best determine whether the margins were clear. If not clear on initial exam, we would go back and re-excise the exact spot in question. Eventually, we would be told that the excision was complete and that we would either directly close the defect or use an appropriate reconstructive technique. This routine resulted in greatly minimizing recurrences, and we also learned a lot about skin pathology in the process. We were fortunate to have such cooperative colleagues.

However, there were types of basal cell lesions, such as morpheaform type, which were extremely bothersome because of their indistinct borders and their propensity to spread with subdermal extension. We were especially concerned about those lesions near the base of the nasal ala or medial canthus that might be tracking along a deeper plane. This is where Mohs's surgery became very useful. Dr. Mohs, a surgeon at the University of Wisconsin, proposed and practiced a method of tissue fixation (with zinc chloride paste). He then removed the fixed specimen, mapping the entire specimen and sectioning in such a way as to determine the adequacy of excision. Dr. William Taylor, a professor of dermatology at

UM and a close friend of Dr. Dingman's, became quite a proponent of this technique. A training program was begun in dermatology, and soon, there were more Mohs surgeons available. In the early days, the procedure often took more than one day, which was a disadvantage for the patients. Eventually, the fresh technique evolved that allowed multiple sections to be examined in a single day. When the completed Mohs procedure provided assurance that the excision was complete, the surgeon could proceed with reconstruction without fear of camouflaging a recurrence and minimizing morbidity time for the patient.

## Treatment of Cutaneous Vascular Lesions

In 1977, Dr. Grabb, with Dr. Malcolm (Biff) MacCollum (1973–75) and Nick Tan, published in PRS the UM's experience with the use dermal tattooing in camouflaging cutaneous hemangiomas (port-wine stains).[30] An attempt was made to reaffirm successful results in a previous study from Toronto. Nineteen children up to sixteen years of age who had tattooing of the congenital port-wine hemangiomas were included in the report. A careful attempt was made to match the tattoo pigment with individual skin tones of each patient. This effort was supervised by Nick Tan, from medical illustration, who had training in preparing and mixing these pigments. None of the patients had ultimate improvement beyond 50 percent after at least two and sometimes five treatments. The consensus of the authors was that this technique was not effective enough in this age group of patients, due in part to gradual leaching out of the pigment.

In 1984, Marks, Argenta, and ROD presented five cases of traumatic arteriovenous malformations of the external carotid system.[31] In the cases presented, the lesions were characterized as containing multiple endothelial-lined channels between the arterial and venous system. The etiology was discussed. Accurate diagnosis is important and often can be made by feeling a thrill on palpation or a bruit on auscultation, and by Doppler study. Unless the lesion is small and well localized, its extent and the specific feeder vessels are best evaluated by arteriography. Four of the five cases presented confirmed by history that inadequate excision leads to recurrence and perhaps significant cosmetic deformity. Complete excision and ligation of all feeder arterial vessels is essential, and long-term follow-up in these five cases revealed no recurrence. Significant defects can result from excision that may require reconstruction. A thorough description of the cases was provided along with an excellent review of the literature. In that same year, Krystyna Pasyk, MD; Dingman; Argenta; and Gary Sandall (pediatric ophthalmologist) reported on eyelid and orbital capillary hemangiomas.[32] Congenital capillary (strawberry) hemangiomas are usually present at birth or shortly thereafter. They go through a growth phase and ultimately spontaneously regress or disappear starting by age five or six. However, those that involve the orbital area and obstruct the vision can result in a variety of ocular problems including loss of vision (amblyopia). The article stressed the critical importance of close coordinated follow-up by a pediatrician, ophthalmologist, and plastic surgeon. Treatment must be started aggressively if the lesion enlarges enough to even partially obstruct the infant's vision. If the visual field becomes totally obstructed, intervention must be carried out within one week to prevent amblyopia. Initially, injectable steroids can be tried, but if not effective in quickly shrinking the tumor, surgical excision must be done. Because these lesions do spontaneously regress, total extirpation is not indicated. Clearing the field of vision is the primary objective.

## *Skin Flaps*

Beginning in 1966, there was a concerted effort both in the laboratory and clinically to study how to improve the efficiency and utility of skin flaps to close wounds. The struggle to successfully close difficult wounds was an ongoing problem for all of us. We were motivated by clinical necessity to find ways to enhance the blood supply to random skin flaps and to find new ways to approach this problem. Time was spent in studying the delay phenomena and exploring various ideas to enhance the vascularity of both random and axial patterned flaps. Examples are the research projects that fellow resident Bob Knode, Bill Grabb, and I contributed to in the VA laboratory in 1966–67.[33,34] Although we were optimistic at the onset, the results unfortunately showed that IV dextran did not enhance the vascularity of either variety of flap in the pig.

Many of the types of flaps available clinically to us at the time were cumbersome and not always successful. I think back to the necessity of applying cross-leg flaps to avulsion injuries of the opposite lower leg and the morbidity from the necessary immobilization. This was described very well in a paper by Grabb, Don Greer, and Bob Wilensky[35] along with Don Greer's chapter in Grabb and Myers' book on flaps.[36]

Dr. Grabb's interests in skin flaps were wide-ranging and sustained. He became familiar with all the centers and surgeons who were working in this extensive and fascinating field of endeavor. The effort culminated in the publication of the book *Skin Flaps*[37] in 1975 that Dr. Grabb edited with Dr. Bert Myers, professor of surgery at Louisiana State University (LSU) and a tireless collaborator in flap research. Dr. Frank McDowell, the editor-in-chief of *PRS*, wrote the foreword for the book. A quote from the foreword clearly stated the book's importance: "For too long we have not had a book devoted to all aspects of all kinds of flaps.

To obtain such information one had to read parts of many books and many papers. Now it is all available to us in a compact volume, both experimental and clinical, written by the leading workers in each phase in the United States and abroad. Herein will be the answer to most of our questions about flaps. And from this we will get ideas for new uses of flaps and a better ways of moving flaps. How fortunate we are."[38] Quotes from the preface, written by Drs. Grabb and Myers, clearly delineated the up-to-date status of the research and clinical development in the field of skin flaps as of the time of publication: "The principles that have been used in planning a skin flap were developed empirically over a period of centuries. In the past decade great advances as a result have permitted us to proceed with more confidence of success in the clinical use of skin flaps. These advances have been the stimulus for this book."[39] There were two major divisions in the text. The first ten chapters pertained to some of the recent research on skin flaps. These chapters included flap circulation as well as effects of anesthetic agents and hyperbaric oxygen. The mechanism of the delay phenomenon, including the role of arteriovenous connections, was also discussed. A summary of the anatomy of cutaneous circulation was also presented. Pioneering authors included, among others, John Reinisch, Rollin Daniel, and Bert Myers, and references to Stuart Milton, a flap research pioneer, who had recently died and to whom the book was dedicated, were also present in the book. He was a close friend of Bill Grabb's and a welcome visitor in Ann Arbor. He was initially responsible for questioning the validity of the absoluteness of length-width ratio in skin flap design.[40]

Continuing from the preface,

> The remaining 31 chapters are devoted to the clinical aspects of skin flaps. In the clinical use of skin flaps, we are moving toward an atlas of safe skin flaps, but there is no rule or formula by which we can design a flap with assurance that it will survive. Rather we must rely on our accumulated experience to know that a flap with its base in a certain place when it's designed to be of so many centimeters in length and a certain number of centimeters in width. In Part II we have asked the contributing authors to orient descriptions of specific flaps according to anatomic landmarks and provide, in centimeters, the dimensions of length and width that, in their experience would assure a viable flap in the healthy adult.[41]

Part II was an inclusive group of chapters providing a clear description of all the known flaps available for defects, literally from head to toe, written by experts recruited by the editors from around the world who had actually used these flaps. It was clearly a masterful accomplishment for its time, and it was the model for the book *Encyclopedia of Flaps*, which Dr. Grabb was working on at the time of his death in 1982. It was published posthumously in 1990[42] and is now in three volumes.

More from the Grabb and Myers preface: "The early determination of blood supply to random pattern and axial pattern flaps deserve emphasis and it was explained that in the clinical situation, one can accurately determine the adequacy of blood supply to both random and axial pattern flaps by the intravenous injection of fluorescein followed by a visualization of the fluorescence under an ultra violet lamp. In an axial pattern flap, a hand-held Doppler flowmeter can help locate and then monitor blood flow in the artery supplying the flap."[43] Some of this experimental work was carried out at UM in clinical studies by Dr. Grabb with Dr. Sigurdur (Siggy) E. Thorvaldsson (1971–73), published in 1974.[44] It was a report of nineteen patients and showed that the use of IV fluorescein at the time of operation was a reliable and safe method for predicting how much of a skin flap would survive after raising it from its normal anatomic location. The results of this study and others as discussed by Dr. Bert Myers, in chapter one in the book *Skin Flaps*, gave us confidence in the reliability of the technique. Based on this study, we began to intraoperatively excise portions of skin flaps that failed to fluoresce. We followed this procedure both with reconstructive flaps and surgical ones such as in prophylactic mastectomies. This technique was a precursor to the currently used "SPY" intraoperative flap monitor.[45] Grabb and Myers' book, *Skin Flaps*, was the bridge between the era of the pioneering understanding of random and axial flaps and the widespread use of musculocutaneous and fasciocutaneous flaps in the coming years.

## *Myocutaneous (Musculocutaneous) Flaps*

The next dramatic steps with understanding flaps were recounted by Leonard Furlow, who with John McCraw coauthored the last chapter describing the dorsalis pedis arterial flap in Grabb and Myers' book. In a 2014 editorial posted in the *Annals of Plastic Surgery*, titled "When Our Vocabulary Changed,"[46] Dr. Furlow explained that before the mid-1970s, the language we plastic surgeons used when we talked about flaps was geometric—length-width ratio, advancement, transposition—or anatomic—cross-leg, abdominal, or temporal, delayed or staged. Flaps, moved in a random network of vessels, often required delay or staging to improve the blood supply or to induce the flap to survive on a reduced blood supply. The few axial flaps previously identified, such as the forehead flap, deltopectoral flap, and neurovascular island flaps in the hand, had very circumscribed uses. The very innovative Dr. Miguel Orticochea reported constructing a penis using a muscle carried on its axial vessels with the overlying skin supplied by perforating vessels from the muscle. Stimulated by that specific solution, John McCraw saw the tremendous potential in understanding and describing a general myocutaneous pattern for the solution of a wide range of reconstructive challenges. When at Emory University, under Dr. Jurkiewicz, Dr. McCraw began defining by dissection a variety of these flaps and, with that knowledge, produced a virtual revolution that changed the field of reconstructive surgery forever.[47] Ultimately, this led Drs. McCraw and P. G. Arnold to begin an annual flap dissection course in 1977 in Norfolk, Virginia, and ultimately to publish McGraw and Arnold's *Atlas of Muscle and Myocutaneous Flaps* in 1980.[48]

As is true with a great many revolutionary advances, there is often a simultaneity leading to wider dissemination of the basic concepts. This was certainly true in the case of the advent of myocutaneous flap concepts in promoting the better understanding of the importance of these flaps for a host of reconstructive problems. Two important articles were published in the same year in *PRS*; the first was by Mathes, Vasconez, and Jurkiewicz, titled "Extensions and Further Application of Muscle Flap Transposition," in 1977.[49] A little later, in the same volume, McCraw, Dibble, and Carraway published "Clinical Definition of Independent Myocutaneous Vascular Territories."[50] Mathes and Nahai published their book, *The Clinical Atlas of Muscle and Musculocutaneous Flaps* in 1979.[51]

Within the UM program, there was a sense of being alert to new ideas from national meetings, specialized conferences, personal conversations and bringing them back to Ann Arbor. The importance of this concept was actively supported by both Dr. Dingman and Dr. Grabb. One practical result of this policy was illustrated by the fact that Larry Berkowitz, a junior resident in 1977, went to the first myocutaneous flap dissection course in Norfolk, Virginia, put on by Dr. McCraw. Larry came back and discussed these new concepts with Paul Izenberg, then his senior resident. They discussed these exciting ideas with Dr. Grabb who enthusiastically encouraged them to clearly define the detailed vascular anatomy of all these flaps. Dr. Paul Izenberg recalled, "Little did we know how much this would change the face of all reconstructive surgery. So off we trundled one evening to the cadaver lab and obtained two to three full fresh cadavers. We outlined and prosected ten to fifteen flaps Larry had seen at the meeting including vessels, landmarks, and surrounding anatomy. The entire plastic surgery section showed up a day later for a teaching section. The fun part was that over the remainder of our residency, the residents became the experts on these flaps, helping each other and changing the face of pressure sore surgery and defect closure."[52] These fresh cadaver dissections were an important advance in the study of surgical anatomy. As mentioned before, no longer were we restricted to the use of embalmed (preserved) cadaver specimens. The availability of these unembalmed anatomic specimens allowed much more precise and detailed dissections especially of small muscles, nerves, and blood vessels. Paul and Larry ultimately defined the anatomy of all the flaps that subsequently entered common usage for a wide variety of reconstructive procedures, including trauma, decubitus ulcers, and reconstruction after cancer resections. These musculocutaneous flaps studied at the time included the gracilis, the tensor fascia lata (TFL), latissimus dorsi, the pectoralis major, the gluteus maximus, the vastus lateralis, and the gastrocnemius. This endeavor led to a much better understanding of differences in patterns in vascular anatomy, which ultimately led to a use of free flaps using direct microvascular transfer. Paul emphasized, "The Section of Plastic Surgery had a great relationship with the Anatomy Department and more importantly, there was no issue getting fresh cadavers for prosection for teaching or individual preparation for surgery. The deaner Bob always had things ready."[53] We were indebted to the UM gross anatomy department for their willing cooperation in providing the anatomic specimens for our plastic surgery education program through their highly respected anatomic donation program.

## *Treatment of Decubitus Ulcers*

Dr. Paul Izenberg recalled that the availability and reliability of the myocutaneous flap changed the residents' attitude toward the surgical treatment of these challenging problems. It turned the treatment of these pressure sores into a fascinating exercise to define the best flap and an enjoyable exercise in anatomical dissections to achieve a successful result. Paul recounted, "The surgery on pressure sores which as random or delayed flaps was always a chore. We used to say with the random flaps the weakest part of the flap, the tip, was the most crucial part of the flap, this failure to get a healed wound was not rare. But then it became 'fun' for us making it an anatomical challenge with a much better chance of the flap surviving exactly where we needed it! That was a real change from what had gone before."[54]

It was emphasized to all of us that the most important aspect of preventing these problems in spinal cord–injured patients was the physical therapy teaching about the physical and social changes needed to avoid the pressure injury in the first place as well as avoiding postoperative recurrences.

In the plastic surgery 1972–73 annual report, it is noted that a research project was set up to be directed by Dr. Jim Norris (resident, 1973–74) to evaluate the results of surgical treatment of patients at UM from 1961 to 1971.[55] The objective was to study the rate and reasons for recurrence after surgery, estimate the cost of treatment, and attempt to ascertain the best nursing and surgical care for these patients. In addition, it was decided as a policy to limit decubitus ulcer patients to four on the plastic surgery service at any one time. Dr. Norris (in a letter to me) said, in effect,

> The study was intended as an accurate record of all pressure sore cases to determine what factors contributed to complications to apply for a study to investigate the feasibility of a spinal cord center in the state of Michigan. Dr. Dingman was most supportive, but even so we got no response from the numbers of organizations that were contacted. Dr. Dingman was deeply concerned about the treatment of all illnesses. When I told him that I would like to do more for the spinal cord injury patients, he gave me his full support. I have sent to you a paper that was presented at the Annual Residents Conference in 1974. It is entitled, "Pressure sores there must be a better way." This paper was never published but it demonstrates the kind of support Dr. Dingman gave me. We felt that the treatment of patients with spinal cord injuries demanded special facilities and felt that the University of Michigan Medical Center should have a spinal cord injury center. Dr. Dingman secured probably the second air fluidized bed produced. We set up a small unit and we wrote letters to a number of foundations asking for support for a spinal cord unit. Incidentally, we had the full support of the administration, the neurosurgical service, and rehabilitation medicine service.[56]

It is interesting to peruse Dr. Dingman's thoughts on the overall management of these difficult patients in the era 1973–74 in the section's annual report from that year:

> We are continuing the study of the etiology and the treatment of pressure sores. Various modalities of treatment such as [random] flaps are being evaluated for their efficacy and complications. Further, various types of pressure relieving beds such as air-fluidized beds as well as the water mattress are being evaluated. These patients continue to present an ongoing serious problem and are in great need of multispecialty care. Our department continues to feel that a cord-injury center would be the most efficient way of utilizing available funds. The average hospitalization of these patients continues to be extensive and the surgical therapy of these sores is one small portion of these cases. Rehabilitation remains the paramount problem and prevention is unquestionably the best mode of therapy for pressure sores.[57]

Fortunately, the advent of seat "cushion" technology and pressure relief with flotation and airbeds became available—their near universal usage has dramatically helped reduce the incidence of these lesions while also avoiding postoperative recurrence.

## *Clinical Microvascular Surgery*

John Markley, our "go-to guy" in this area, reports on the development of clinical microsurgery in Ann Arbor:

> In 1970, during my Stanford residency six-month lab rotation, I taught myself microvascular technique in the empty but still equipped micro lab Harry Buncke left behind when he left Stanford. I visited him a couple times at his lab in Mountain View, and used some written material he had generated, and just taught myself, doing rat kidney transplants, end-end arterial, venous, and ureteral anastomoses. This led to doing a rat renal transplant immunologic study with the transplant surgeon at Stanford (Lucas) which was published in 1970. In 1974, I returned to Ann Arbor, and used ENT monocular scopes for some nerve repairs at UM and SJMH. In February 1976, I performed the first digital replant in the state of Michigan, at SJMH, using monocular ENT scope, for a 12-year-old girl's thumb, which was successful. Several months later, I performed the first digital replant at UM, using monocular ENT scope, on a two-year-old's thumb (!), which was successful too. This publicity led to more patients in the hand clinic, 1977–78. Although there was by now a binocular scope in the Sargent Lab in Kresge, there was still no binocular scope in the UM ORs. For the next few replants, I had to roll the lab scope through several buildings, two elevators, to either Mott or Main OR to do the emergency cases, often alone in the middle of the night. The vibration from this started to damage the scope and I threatened to stop doing replants unless the hospital bought at least one for an OR. Dr. Turcotte came through with one for Mott, and eventually for the main OR, in late 1978 or early 1979. Replants done in 1976–80 were seventeen digits (sixteen patients) replanted or revascularized by me with resident assistance, one failure, and 94% success. I did some more in 1981–83 also, but don't have the records for some reason.
> From 1978–83, there were elective microsurgical tissue transfers, toe to hand, fibular bone grafts, quite a few free flaps and then micronerve and microvascular muscle flaps for facial paralysis—in addition to the replants, I did elective microsurgical reconstruction during this period at the university, including several toe-to-hand

transfers, one or two free microvascular fibular bone grafts, and quite a few free flaps of various sorts. During the same period (1978–83), I did fifteen clinical human facial paralysis reconstructions with various combinations of free graft, transposed muscle flap, and microvascular free muscle flap, all re-innervated by cross-face facial nerve grafts. I had the confidence to do this based on prior clinical work done by others and on the Faulkner/Markley experience, and indeed was rewarded with reasonable clinical improvement in most of these patients (see pp. 40–4—most of the UM plastic surgery residents in this time period were involved in these cases).

Dr. Markley continued, "In 1983, I got together with Dr. Dingman, Jerry Turcotte, Chairman of Surgery, Robert Bartlett, General Surgery, and Dr. William Smith, the head of Orthopedics, to organize a formal replant service for the University of Michigan. Tom Stevenson who had just joined Plastic Surgery, being appointed by Dr. Grabb before he died, became the director of this joint activity between Plastic Surgery, Orthopedic Surgery, and General Surgery."[58]

For the residents, the combination of Dr. Markley's superb microvascular training, the invaluable experience they gained in Dr. Acland's training program in Louisville (see p. 73), and the personal practice time that they had the opportunity for in the Sargent laboratory provided them with excellent preparation to respond to emergency demands such as major extremity traumatic amputations. Dr. Ernie Manders (1979–81) recounted,

> We became fine surgeons fast—because we had to BE the surgeon. One example comes to mind to provide contrast for today's residency. I was on call and a child came in with his foot cut off at the ankle. There was just the most tenuous of skin bridges left, with all major structures divided. I called up fellow resident Mike Watanabe and asked if he would like to help me replant the foot. Sure he said. So we called our staff Lou Argenta and told him what we planned. "Call me if you need me," he replied. We succeeded and the next few days were a whirlwind of publicity. The child's picture was on the front page of the Ann Arbor News and Mike and I were called by a local radio station for comments on air. We had our fifteen minutes of fame.[59]

Dr. Bob Gilman (1980–82) recently brought to our attention another dramatic case, the details of which follow:

> In February of 1982, the first complete replantation of an amputated hand was accomplished at the UM on the plastic surgery service.

A twenty-three-year-old male had sustained a complete amputation of his left hand just above the wrist in an industrial saw accident. The patient had been transferred to the UM from Monroe, Michigan, after he had received emergency care. In the OR, Dr. Gilman and Dr. Gordon Derman, the senior and junior residents on call, dissected the ends of the blood vessels, nerves, and tendons from the cut end of the amputated hand. At the same time, Dr. Louis Argenta, then a faculty staff member, and Dr. Malcolm Marks, another senior resident, dissected the corresponding structures on the cut end of the stump of the patient's arm. An orthopedic team plated the radius and ulna after slightly shortening the bones to reduce tension on the subsequent vascular repairs. Then the four-man plastic surgery team repaired an artery and two veins. Once circulation to the hand had been successfully established, the second artery and the nerves and tendons were repaired. The patient's hand survived, and gained protective sensation and enough motion for use as an assisting hand.[60]

As Dr. Izenberg added,

Cases like these partial and complete replantations as well as reconstructions with microvascular tissue transfer have literally become routine since those early beginnings.[61]

## Shotgun Injuries to the Face

This was one horrifying and extremely difficult group of patients. The vast majority represented unsuccessful suicide attempts, in which the initial air release from the barrel of the gun in the mouth kicks forward and the main injury is to the midface and jaws. So the patients not only had acute massive wounds but they were also in need of both prolonged reconstruction and psychiatric care. Prior to the era of myocutaneous flaps and free tissue transfer, the reconstructive options were often carried out over several years. These patients' names remained imprinted in the residents' memories, and often, as they gathered at meetings, they would say to each other "... do you remember Harvey so and so ..." and recall how one may have done the initial debridement, another a tube flap transfer, and yet a third a bone graft. Reconstructive tools such as a forehead or deltopectoral flap were often inadequate to compensate for the three-dimensional aspects of these complex and massive wounds. The patients were often left having to wear a mask and carry a towel at all times. It was not until the early 1980s that the new reconstructive advances allowed reasonable reconstruction for these desperate patients. As Dr. Izenberg shared, "Still the results with so much tissue missing was always limiting. Hopefully preventive psychiatric care will reduce these horrendous injuries. Face transplant surgery, as it evolves, may also provide more comprehensive reconstruction possibilities."[62]

## Gender Reassignment Surgery

Sometime in the late 1960s, a conference was organized at the request of a UM staff psychiatrist to discuss treatment of transgender patients who had sought care at the university hospital. It was pointed out to us that understanding of transsexualism had progressed to its being considered a specific disease entity and a well-defined diagnosis in the psychiatric literature. The psychiatrist explained that it was a unique condition and not a variant of homosexuality. We were also told that there was no effective or perhaps even justified medical or psychiatric treatment. The current thinking was that, in selected patients, hormonal management and gender reassignment surgery was the best option. Consequently, a team was set up comprising specialists from relevant disciplines, including psychiatry (Dr. Joseph Pearson), psychology testing (Dr. Richard Hertel, PhD), social work, urology (Dr. Joseph Cerny), gynecology/endocrine (Drs. Bob Jaffee and George Morley), and plastic surgery (Drs. Grabb and myself). All potential patients were evaluated by psychiatry, underwent psychological testing, and had a social work evaluation. Additional requirements included cross-dressing as the sex they wished to be, appropriate hormonal therapy, and having lived as a transsexual for up to two years. If successful in these endeavors, then the patients were reevaluated and were required to be accepted as surgical candidates by the entire team. One technique I employed in my evaluation was to see the patient with a medical student who would be unaware of the patient's condition. If the patient was convincing in manner and appearance to the student, this was an important factor in my final approval. The vast majority of our patients were males wanting to be females and had insurance coverage through the Detroit auto companies where they worked. In general, following surgery, they were usually quite satisfied with their conversion. At the time, we were lining the neo-vagina with skin grafts and contractures in these reconstructions created need for prolonged follow-up for the gynecologists who were the primary caregivers in the follow-up period. This situation eventually led to termination of the program. The female to male patients were more difficult, at that time, as we were limited for penile reconstruction to using delayed, multistaged abdominal tube flaps with an internal lumen for the urethra. The results were less than ideal and tedious for both the patient and surgeon. Even with the limitations and complications, the majority of these transsexual patients were grateful for the team's sympathetic understanding of their condition and our willingness to be involved in their care. For a variety of reasons, the program was not ultimately sustainable. It was certainly a unique educational experience for us to have a better understanding of this newly described and, in general, poorly understood condition. Newer techniques and more psychological understanding have helped these programs to flourish again within the UM plastic surgery section under Dr. William Kuzon.

## *Clinical Skin Expansion*

Dr. Eric Austad had the most intimate recollections of the program from its inception at the UM:

> In one of our occasional conversations over his later years, Radovan recalled to me his initial conversation with implant manufacturer Rudy Schulte, in which he outlined his concept of a tissue expander while driving Schulte to a local airport in the fall of 1975. Driving guests was a universal resident function in the 1970s. Schulte was impressed, and a few months later Radovan received his first expander. It was a two-tubed balloon which allowed inflation or deflation as desired, and his patient presented a particularly difficult problem: a large diabetic foot ulcer which he successfully treated with an expanded cross-leg flap at a local Veterans' Hospital. As a failure of this rather heroic first procedure would have been a significant setback, Radovan's confidence and/or luck was remarkable.
>
> In October of 1976, our Section Chairman, Bill Grabb, attended the American Society of Plastic and Reconstructive Surgery (ASPRS) meeting in Boston and returned with the news that a California plastic surgeon had presented a "poster session" describing his work with early versions of what became known as the "Radovan Expander." This was my first knowledge of Radovan's work and I wrote him a letter on the university letterhead inviting some interplay of our mutual interests, but got no response. In the meantime, guinea pigs became our basic model for animal work with self-inflating expanders, as no one had actually studied or reported any information regarding the basic safety of the expansion process. Specifically, was this a safe procedure? What cellular changes occurred? Was vascularity compromised? What happened to hair follicles? Was mitosis stimulated or was "malignant transformation" induced? What happened to nerves? In general, did expansion result in useful and safe tissue? We believed, in contrast to Radovan, that these questions had to be addressed before we could consider human trials. In summary, we went first to the laboratory, while Radovan went first to his local V.A.

By the early 1980s, Radovan's implant became available on a limited basis and other Michigan residents became very involved in the clinical use of expanders. Lou Argenta gained extensive experience with the Radovan expanders, particularly in the head, neck, and breast, and he went on to become a world-class authority on expansion. Ernie Manders presented outstanding results using expanders in nasal reconstruction, electrifying the attendees of the first national tissue expansion symposium sponsored by our section and the Educational Foundation of the ASPRS in May of 1981. In his demonstration of the intricate folds involved, he used his necktie unforgettably. He also went on to become internationally known for his work with expansion and developed and marketed the "croissant expander" and the "differential expander," which are particularly useful for breast and scalp reconstruction. I chaired that meeting, where Drs. George Cherry, Krystyna Pasyk, Malcolm Marks, and Ken McClatchey all presented both laboratory and clinical work, and both Dr. Radovan and Dr. Gordon Sasaki reviewed their clinical experience. (Dr. Sasaki later wrote a classic textbook on expansion and lectured on its use internationally.) Lou Argenta and I were invited to write the chapter on expansion for McCarthy's *Plastic Surgery*, the eight-volume successor to Converse's book. In February of 1984, Rod Rohrich organized the first international tissue expansion symposium at Oxford, and invited virtually all of the major workers in the field to a most-successful two-day event. Many subsequent courses and symposia followed.

As a final note, I would express my gratitude to Dr. William C. Grabb, my mentor and friend, my fellow residents and staff, and the colleagues worldwide who have helped, challenged, and encouraged my work. If I had not had the privilege of working in Dr. G. Barry Pierce's lab as an undergraduate, where I first saw and used semipermeable membranes, and if I never had the experience of observing the sequelae of massive weight loss as a resident at Michigan, I would have missed this entire adventure.[63]

In 1984, along with Drs. Rohrich and Izenberg, I published a case demonstrating the usefulness of skin expansion during reconstruction of the upper two-thirds of the external ear.[64] The expansion facilitated draping of the otherwise insufficient superior retro-auricular skin over the autogenous costal cartilage framework of the reconstruction. This is a good example of one of the many types of deformities where expansion was being use for distinct advantage.

## Breast Surgery

*1. Reduction Mammoplasty*

Reduction mammoplasty was a common operation early in the program. The operation described by Strombeck[65] was the procedure of choice. The technique consisted of the Wise pattern reduction with a horizontal pedicle containing the nipple-areolar complex on the retained breast tissue. As we gained more experience, particularly in reduction of larger breasts, the ease and safety in repositioning of the nipple-areolar complex seemed unreliable. Ron Wexler learned about the McKissock vertical pedicle technique[66] at the 1971 Montreal ASPRS meeting. We discussed it and together did the first case in Michigan and were impressed that the vertical mobility of the pedicle seemed to overcome some of the disadvantages of the Strombeck technique. However, the narrowness of the pedicle and the question of reliability of the vascularity and sensation to the nipple-areolar complex in larger and more ptotic breasts concerned us. When Drs. Courtiss and Goldwyn described the inferior pedicle technique in 1977,[67] it seemed the perfect answer for the types of breasts that might require maximum vertical repositioning of the nipple-areolar complex. Gaining experience in this technique confirmed our initial enthusiasm. In more pendulous and larger breasts, necessitating longer pedicles, we learned the vascularity of the pedicle could be enhanced by designing the base of the pedicle along the entire width of the inframammary fold. Because of the flexibility of this procedure for any size and shape of breast, the mobility of the pedicle, and a greater sense of vascular security, the inferior pedicle technique became the standard procedure for almost all of our reductions. An early exception to the use of inferior-pedicled reductions were high-risk patients with large breasts in whom we wanted to avoid any significant blood loss and who seemed to be well suited for the amputation-free nipple technique. The not-so-infrequent hypertrophic scars in the lateral extent of the inframammary scar were the main disadvantage of reductions using the Wise pattern, particularly in younger patients. Ultimately, this led to a search for procedures with a shorter horizontal scar, which have become more common.

In planning for reductions and ptosis correction, there was always discussion about the proper positioning of the new nipple during preoperative measurements. In an effort to establish better criteria for the ideal nipple placement relative to breast size, together with Mr. Denis Lee of medical sculpture and Art Rathjen from the Dow Corning Company, we proposed a clinical study to clarify this issue. Art was interested in getting accurate measurements of normal, attractive breasts of various sizes to help with Dow Corning's design for external prosthesis, while Denis was an artist and sculptor, knowledgeable about artistic proportions. Because of my interest in surgical solutions, the most significant measurement for me was the ideal distance from the sternal notch to the nipple in the postoperative breast. We recruited a group of young, female university students who felt they had "normal" breasts and volunteered for the study and underwent measurements and photographs of their breast size and position. The subjects' breast size varied in bra size from 32 to 38 and cup sizes from B to D. The study documented that the nipple distance was longer with progressive increase in bra size and also increased by cup size. We arbitrarily chose C-cup breast size, which we felt was a reasonable postoperative endpoint for most reduction patients. We discovered that for bra size C cup, the distance averaged almost 21 cm for 32C, 22.5 cm for 34C, almost 24 cm for 36C, and slightly over 25 cm for 38C. This concept was supported by the update Courtiss and Goldwyn reported in 1980 where they also discussed concern about placing the nipple-areolar complex too high.[68] So the usual recommended 22 cm preoperative measurement was too short for many patients. In addition, we learned to take into account the individual patient's breast skin elasticity and the postoperative effect on planned nipple-areolar position. I am convinced that this study helped us to plan breast reduction so that the nipple-areolar complex was not too high, which, should it occur, was almost impossible to satisfactorily correct. This was also helpful in preoperative planning for breast ptosis patients. A breakthrough in breast ptosis correction was provided by Dr. Daniel Marchac, from France, when he demonstrated the importance in reshaping the breast by splitting the lower pole of the gland up to the areola, and then overlapping the two segments horizontally so that the final improvement in shape and position was not just dependent on the skin reshaping but could be achieved by restructuring the breast tissue.[69]

### 2. Breast Augmentation

The first Dow Corning gel implants, which contained viscous silicone gel of various viscosities within a silicone (Silastic) envelope, became available in 1964 (after a report by Cronin and Gerow from the University of Texas[70]). Many of the previous nonautologous materials used in attempted augmentations had resulted in serious complications and required removal. This included injected free silicone, much of which was not always of medical grade leading to serious complications. The new silicone implants were thick walled and contained quite viscous gel. They were designed with Dacron patches on the back to stimulate fixation. Originally, they were placed in a subglandular position through inframammary incisions. As an alternative to using absorbable dermal sutures in closing these incisions, which often resulted in suture reactions and delayed wound healing, we introduced a double layer removable subcuticular permanent nylon suture closure, running both in the deep dermal layer and the epidermal layer. This technique insured much reduced possibility of suture reactions and significantly lessened concern of possible extrusion of the implant. Saline-filled implants were also available but were of somewhat limited popularity because both patients and surgeons feared deflation. This potential was greatly reduced by the posterior flap valve being replaced by an anterior-placed injection valve. Early replacement with a new implant after deflation was important to avoid contracture of the existing implant pocket. Spontaneous deflation was actually quite uncommon, and considering the worry arising later regarding the safety of silicone gel, it would have been wiser if we had used them more frequently. Capsular contractures were common with the gel implants (somewhat less with saline filled) and manual "cracking" (putting external pressure of the breast to force the capsular tissue to rupture and allow the implant to relax) became a common office procedure. In the early years following the introduction of gel implants, one manufacturer tried to alleviate the unnatural feel by making a thinner shell and a more liquid gel. As a result, with closed capsulotomy, there was a possibility of extrusion of gel into the adjacent tissues or into an axillary lymph node, a case of which I reported in *PRS* in 1979.[71] Gel bleed through the implant shell also became more of a problem.

One of the early clinical research projects we carried out in the late 1960s was a psychological evaluation of preoperative augmentation patients in conjunction with two psychiatric colleagues. The work was not published but the analysis of over thirty female patients in their third decade revealed that the vast majority seeking augmentation did not manifest any serious psychological problems. We also learned that by using open-ended questions in patient interviews, we gained a lot of information about the patients' deeper feelings about themselves that allowed us to be more understanding in our care of them.

We quickly realized that with augmentation mammoplasty, intraoperative implant selection was impractical. We needed a method whereby we could obtain patient approval of the appropriate implant size preoperatively. The simplest solution we found was for the patient to buy a bra with the proper number for her chest size and the new cup size she wished to be. In the old Jacobson's retail store across the street from our downtown Ann Arbor office in the Tower Plaza, I identified a helpful salesperson who volunteered to advise these patients after I described what we were trying to accomplish and helped them select the appropriate size bra under various styles of clothing. The patient would then bring this new bra to a second office visit. Using available implant sizers in the bra allowed the proper size implant to be selected. Involving the patient in the size selection led to a much greater degree of postoperative patient satisfaction.

Although capsular contractures were not as great a problem with saline implants, we began to try to alter the configuration of the scar tissue contracture by the use of soluble steroids placed in the implant. Dr. Louis Argenta and I reported long-term results in a series of patients with a fairly high dose of the soluble steroids within the implants.[72] The surrounding tissue atrophy leading to implant ptosis in the patients was common but inconsistent. We did not feel that the dosage would necessarily be the only factor. We recommended that even if smaller doses of steroid were used in any prospective research project with saline-filled implants, there should be long-term follow-up. Some of these adverse effects did not appear for several months or even for more than a year after the implant was placed.[73] With a lower dose, it might be an even slower process. Fortunately, in this group of patients, atrophic changes that precipitated the ptosis were reversible following removal of the steroid containing implant. If the implant were replaced with one not containing steroids, we found that we could make a new pocket in the correct position behind the existing one that would lead to a satisfactory result.

Placement of the breast implants under the pectoral muscle had first been described in 1968. The report of one hundred cases by Kenneth Pickrell et al. in 1977[74] as well as presentations at national meetings by Paule Regnault, a Canadian plastic surgeon from Montreal, renewed our interest in that technique. Because of the resulting much lower incidence of capsular contracture, the subpectoral placement became our standard approach. Dr. Thomas Hudak (resident, 1968–70) was our visiting professor in 1980 and shared with all of us his preference and experience with the procedure. He recollected, "I enjoyed my time as the Visiting Clinical Professor (1980) when I taught the residents the technique for submuscular breast implantation, a procedure that when properly done significantly decreased capsule formation. The implants for augmentation were placed submuscular with partial release of the medial attachment of the pectoral muscle. The release of the muscle prevented the implants from being pushed laterally from beneath the muscle."[75]

Once we realized that the normal relationship of the pectoral muscle covered only the upper half of the implant and that the lower part could be placed in an expanded subglandular pocket contiguous with the subpectoral position, we were able to use larger implants that gave a more satisfactory and natural result. The peri-areolar incision, although popular with many, was not, for some of us, convenient in dissecting the subpectoral space. In the case of unmarried women, the transaxillary approach for subpectoral breast augmentation became popular to avoid any chest wall scar. In the mid-1970s, a special subpectoral dissection instrument was designed by Drs. Dingman, Agris, and Wilensky.[76] The latter two were both residents in 1976.

During these years, we enjoyed many advantages of the free exchange of information among plastic surgeons from regional hospitals, such as Providence and Beaumont. New techniques we used included details about transaxillary approach using inflatable implants and the marked advantage of intercostal Marcaine blocks to supplement local anesthesia with sedation. Placing the blocks in the mid-axillary line with small, short needles avoided the incidence of pneumothorax. This combination worked very nicely in outpatient augmentation procedures in an outpatient or office OR setting.

### 3. Prophylactic Mastectomy

In the mid-1970s, there was a renewed concern about the possibility of progression of premalignant breast disease in patients with a maternal history of breast cancer. At SJMH, we formed an interdisciplinary team of general and plastic surgeons, radiologists, and pathologists who met, evaluated the patient, and recommended appropriate treatment. This was at a time before there was knowledge of a high-risk breast cancer gene. There was an ongoing argument about the rationale for prophylactic mastectomy that left a minimal amount of subareolar breast tissue in place even with coring out the nipple versus complete mastectomy. Our impression, at the time, was that the former procedure gave patients considered high risk, and particularly those who had lost family members to breast cancer, considerable peace of mind. Obviously, they required close follow-up by a breast oncologist. To my knowledge, there was no breast cancer that showed up later in any of our patients.

In these prophylactic mastectomy patients, there was always concern about viability of the skin flaps if adequate breast tissue removal was accomplished. The use of low-dosage and slowly injected intravenous fluorescein evaluation proved to be very helpful in determining the viability of the skin flaps and allowing a single-stage reconstruction when indicated (see p. 77).

In 1978, Jarrett et al.[77] reported improved reconstructive results by placing the implant not only subpectoral but also under adjacent portions of the serratus anterior muscle, to create a total submuscular position. This idea was rapidly taken up at Michigan and became the method of choice in this group of patients. In all categories of breast reconstructive patients, complications of implant extrusion and capsular contracture were greatly reduced by placing the implants totally submuscularly, and appearance and patient satisfaction were greatly improved. Another option for autologous reconstruction without implants, particularly in complicated secondary cases, was the transverse rectus abdominis myocutaneous (TRAM) flap (for discussion, see "Breast Reconstruction" section). This could be performed as a bilateral procedure in patients with bilateral prophylactic mastectomies who had unsatisfactory implant reconstruction or for any patients requiring removal of bilateral damaged implants.

## 4. Breast Reconstruction

Early in the program, breast reconstruction did not receive much attention from general surgeons, and there were not many patients requesting it. Dr. Paul Izenberg recounted, "We began with some very basic approaches placing silicone implants under the mastectomy flaps resulting more frequently than not in severe capsular contracture looking like a baseball, being painful, no sense of symmetry, and occasional extrusion. But many of these patients kept the implants as it meant an attempt to return to 'normal.'"[78] The deformity from radical mastectomy, with an absent pectoralis major muscle and often a chest partially covered by a split-thickness skin graft (STSG), was a formidable challenge for reconstructive surgeons. Dr. Izenberg continued, "There was very little that could be done with the radical mastectomy patients at this time or those with severe radiation damage, not an infrequent sequela of the treatment."[79] With the few of these patients on whom we attempted reconstruction, we used either large rotated, delayed flaps or staged abdominal tube flaps, but the results were not satisfactory. As Dr. Izenberg said, "They didn't look good, took a very long time, and there was lots of patient morbidity."[80] When myocutaneous flaps became available, a better option was to transfer the latissimus dorsi myocutaneous flap with a skin island to the anterior chest to provide muscle and skin cover for an implant. Better results were obtained, but not all patients would accept the donor site. Dr. Izenberg observed, "Once modified radical mastectomies became the standard of care, we learned to place the implants under the [preserved] pectorals muscle with the lower one-third covered by external oblique fascia and rectus fascia. Not perfect but better. As mentioned previously, tissue expansion came along with introduction of the Radovan expander [constructed with a separate valve attached with a tube] which caught on quickly and we began using it, elevating some lateral serratus in addition to the pectoralis muscle to help with cover."[81] This was another significant improvement but still required the use of an implant with the potential associated problems with capsular contracture.

In 1982, Paul Izenberg and I became aware of the TRAM flap, which was originally labeled a *transverse island flap*, but was really the *transverse rectus abdominis musculocutaneous* flap, first reported by Hartrampf, Sheflan, and Black in 1982.[82] As we were learning the technique, Paul and I did the first few cases as cosurgeons. We both felt the collaboration was well worthwhile, as together we were able to more efficiently work out many of the technical details of the new and exciting reconstructive procedure. This ushered in a whole new era of breast reconstruction using only autogenous tissue, particularly well suited for breast cancer patients having undergone radiation. With more experience, it became possible to use this as a means of primary reconstruction at the same time as the mastectomy. An added benefit was that the patient also received an abdominoplasty in the process. In 1984, Dr. Roger Friedman, as a senior resident, along with his faculty mentor Dr. Lou Argenta, did one of the first microvascular transfers of a TRAM flap for breast reconstruction, combining the microvascular techniques described by Dr. Markley and knowledge of this new flap design.[83]

Nipple reconstruction became available and could be accomplished in selected cases by sharing a large contralateral nipple-areolar complex.[84] In most cases, however, a small local skin flap to create a nipple combined with tattooing to create the areola was very successful.

During this time, a significant number of patients and providers joined a movement to force insurance companies to cover postmastectomy reconstruction. I had a patient who, with my help, lobbied the Ohio state legislature to mandate insurance coverage. Ohio's passage of this mandate was a step toward subsequent national acceptance for insurance coverage for breast reconstruction and, eventually, for appropriate surgery of the opposite breast by all health insurance companies including Medicare and Medicaid.

## Cleft Lip and Palate

In any discussion on this subject, we must emphasize Bill Grabb's interest and devotion to the field of cleft lip and palate. This is well illustrated by his very comprehensive book, *Cleft Lip and Palate*, published in 1971 with coauthors Sheldon Rosenstein, DDS, professor of orthodontics at Northwestern Dental School, and Kenneth Bzoch, PhD, at the University of Florida.[85] It covered all aspects of the cleft sequence, was very authoritative for its time, and received good reviews. In addition to Dr. Grabb, UM contributors included Dr. Dingman along with Ted Dodenhoff, a resident at the time, with a chapter on surgical correction of mandibular deformities in mature cleft patients. The book also included my contribution of a chapter on oronasal fistulas.

As we mentioned in chapter one, Dr. John Kemper was an early practitioner in the treatment of clefts and beautifully stated the case for the multidisciplinary approach to these patients: "Rehabilitation of the cleft palate patient may be likened to a great drama in which there are a number of actors, each playing an important role under the direction of one individual, the surgeon, who is responsible for its management and production. The most distinguished and important character, the central figure in the play, is the patient, whose successful performance is dependent on the skillful guidance of the director [the surgeon] and the combined efforts of all other members of the cast." In this presentation, he went on to discuss the other critical aspects of care of the cleft patient, including feeding, reassuring the parents that the child will in all probability develop to be a completely normal child, and emphasizing the importance of their continued cooperation in the rehabilitation of the child over a number of years. He also acknowledged the importance of specialized surgical training and achieving not only technical skill but also good surgical judgment. He also stressed the importance of early repair of any lip defect to help mold the displaced alveolar segments, the careful observation for ear infections, and the postsurgical consultation with speech therapists, as well as early institution of active and passive palatal exercises. He closed by stressing that dental care be carried out at the right time and in the right manner including appropriate consultations with a prosthodontist. Finally, he stated the responsibility of the surgeon for timely correction of the commonly associated secondary facial deformities.[86] All of these important aspects taught to us by Drs. Dingman and Grabb formed the basis for our care of the various aspects of the oral cleft deformity. A significant aspect of our care for these children was the financial support available through the generous and well-administered Michigan Crippled Children's fund. This provided total financial support for the comprehensive care of cleft lip and palate patients until eighteen years of age.

*1. Unilateral Cleft Lip (UCL)*

Although there was some pressure by parents and relatives to operate on babies with unilateral clefts as newborns, we felt that it was better to wait until about three months of age. Another rule Dr Grabb insisted upon and we all followed was the 10-10-10 marker: 10 weeks, 10 lb, and 10 gm of hemoglobin. The wait usually assured the baby was healthy but, just as important, that the parents had a chance to bond with the child. We watched the parents go from seeing only the cleft deformity when they looked at their newborn child to seeing, at two to three months of age, a beautiful healthy baby with a limited defect. We came to realize this early bonding of the parents and the cleft baby was essential for the future welfare of the child. Many of our cleft patients were referred from the newborn nursery at SJMH. Our good relationship with the pediatricians facilitated our seeing the patients in the hospital shortly after birth. This allowed us to reassure the family that they could expect that their child would be able to lead a normal life before any discussion of specifics of surgical procedures or speech therapy.

After Dr. Millard published his classic description of the rotation-advancement technique for repair of the UCL in 1964,[87] this became the standard approach that we used at the UM. It worked well for many clefts. However, we began noticing less-than-satisfactory results in creating lip symmetry in the more severe complete unilateral clefts with excessive vertical shortness in the lateral segment. At a UM-sponsored Cleft Lip and Palate conference in the early 1970s, Dr. Ernie Kaplan from Stanford[88] was the first person to propose a modification of the Millard technique for UCL rotation incision when a back cut was required. He proposed making a slightly curved incision directly over to the lower extent of the proposed back cut, thereby avoiding the curved incision extending up to the columellar-labial junction. This concept, together with Dr. Robert Pool's modification of the rotation-advancement technique, made it applicable to all degrees of the UCL deformity. Dr. Pool, from Beaumont Hospital in Michigan, described this approach to us in Ann Arbor in a series of lectures as visiting professor (Photo 54).[89] The two main aspects of this modification were to have the rotation incision on the cleft side be placed slightly below the critically important aesthetic unit of the labial-columellar junction. This distance would increase proportionally to the degree of shortness of the lip on the cleft side and be limited to a maximum of 4 mm. The other important technical aspect was that the upper level of the lateral segment advancement flap was placed below the alar base to the same extent as the medial segment rotation incision was inferior to the columellar-labial junction. This idea was stimulated by his recognition of the difficulty of rotation advancement in cases where the dimensions of the lateral lip segment are deficient.[90] This design allowed the lateral segment, when advanced, to unfold and its vertical height to lengthen. The technique proved to be very adaptable to all variations of severity of the UCL. Dr. Markley, using his well-developed sense of spatial relations and mathematical skills, helped the rest of

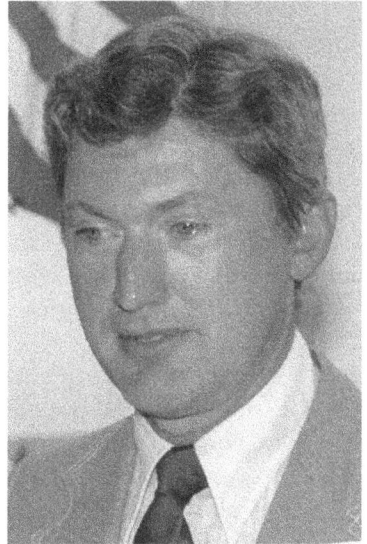

Photo 54: Robert Pool, MD.

us to understand the subtleties of this procedure. After I had experience using it, I became convinced of its amazing versatility in the repair of all varieties of primary unilateral clefts as well as for secondary revisions and was encouraged to continue to use it and also to teach it. I feel very indebted to Dr. Pool for his willingness to share and teach his technique.

## 2. Bilateral Cleft Lip (BCL)

In those early days, as we were one of the few major cleft referral centers in Michigan, we always seemed to have a greater proportion of the more challenging BCL patients compared with UCL patients. A lot of these patients came from the Upper Peninsula of Michigan. They were often referred directly to Drs. Dingman, Grabb, and me both as newborns and as older children. In regard to surgery for BCL, I had an amazing experience at a national meeting when a "light bulb" went off and suddenly I realized that there was a good solution to a previously intractable problem. We all had appreciated how difficult it was to achieve satisfactory aesthetic and functional repair in cases of complete BCLs. Dr. Ralph Millard, at the ASPRS meeting in 1970, presented his idea for unifying the orbicularis muscle from the lateral segments in the midline behind a narrowed prolabium in the primary repair of a BCL. It was published in 1971.[91] The results shown were so striking that there was instantaneous recognition in the audience of how important this modification was. Soon after that meeting, I saw a teenage patient with a typical secondary BCL deformity with orbicularis muscle bulging in the lateral segments and deficient prolabial vermilion. The result of my revising the lip by bringing the muscle together in the midline and using the excess lateral vermillion to replace the previously inadequate and mismatched prolabial vermilion was dramatic. I presented the case at ASPRS, and it was then published in *PRS* in 1974, coauthored by Don Greer and Gary Nobel who were both residents at the time.[92] After seeing the published article, Dr. Millard asked whether he could include a description of the key points of the case with the photographs in his second volume of *Cleft Craft*.[93] I felt much honored by that request. Ultimately, muscle union became a standard feature of both primary and secondary BCL repair at the UM. As described in Millard's 1971 article, we were also banking the "forked flaps" arising from narrowing the lateral edges of the prolabium to later use for lengthening the columella that was almost always too short.

Often, we were confronted with a child with a previously repaired BCL who had a tight and retruded upper lip and a full, redundant lower lip. Shifting a full-thickness Abbe flap on a vascularized vascular pedicle from the lower to the upper lip corrected the imbalance and allowed the insufficient philtral tissue, still attached to the inferior aspect of the columella, to be shifted upward to produce columellar lengthening. An article published in 1971 by Drs. Dingman and Grabb states clearly the difficulty we all came to appreciate about the BCL and palate. As quoted from this article, "Problems of the double cleft are infinitely greater than those exhibited by a single cleft; the difficulties are multiplied several times. The bilateral cleft lip and palate remains one of the most challenging deformities in all of plastic and reconstructive surgery."[94] The article recommended early release of the tethered columella using Millard's "forked flaps," closure of the soft palate between fifteen and twenty-four months, and delaying closure of the hard palate until more complete maxillary growth occurred.

### 3. Cleft Palate

One of the major early advances in the management of cleft palate patients was recognition of the potential for damage to the middle ear caused by dysfunction of the Eustachian tubes in infants and young children. In collaboration with our ENT colleagues, we instituted prophylactic treatment in all cleft palate patients either when the associated cleft lip was repaired or when an isolated cleft palate was repaired at about one year of age. Myringotomy was performed, fluid removed, and a small silastic tube inserted to allow equalization of pressure in the middle ear through the eardrum, thereby bypassing the dysfunctional Eustachian tube. Avoiding hearing loss was especially important in cleft patients learning speech. With growth and palatal closure, eventually the tube could be discontinued in the older child once normal Eustachian function developed.

As far as the actual palate repair was concerned, we were forever trying to find the correct balance to achieve acceptable speech and avoid maxillary growth disturbance, and through these years, it was an ongoing process. The operative visualization and the surgical access to these frequently demanding repairs were greatly facilitated by the availability of the famous and widely used Dingman mouth gag (Photo 55).[95] The mouth gag was formulated and manufactured by Richard Sarns of

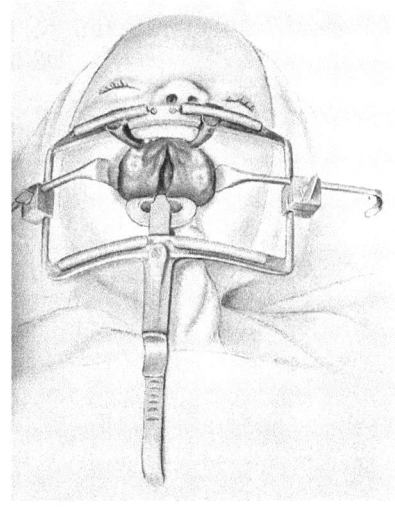

*Photo 55:* The Dingman mouth gag, showing the exposure of the operative field as a result of its proper placement in a young cleft palate patient.

the Sarns Inc. engineering firm in Ann Arbor, Michigan. Mr. Sarns told me that Dr. Dingman had invited him into the OR to visualize the need for improved instrumentation to increase safe cleft palate operative exposure as well as to minimize the necessity for unnecessary assistants around a very small operative field.[96] Sarns designed a multipurpose instrument on a square frame that met four essential requirements: adjustable tongue depressors to stabilize the endotracheal tube as well as the patient's tongue; provide a secure, as well as anatomically safe, open mouth position; lateral cheek retraction; and tightly coiled small springs attached to the upper and lower horizontal bar to hold multiple suture lengths after they had been tied in place to allow them all to be trimmed in a single maneuver. Three different sizes of tongue depressors were made available to allow the instrument to be used in all ages of cleft patients. This well-designed instrument quickly became an essential mainstay for all types of cleft palate surgery and is now in worldwide use.

The idea of closing the soft palate first, allowing the hard palate cleft to narrow, and delaying hard palate closure until eruption of the primary first molar at around thirteen to nineteen months was very appealing for minimizing potential for palatal narrowing except for the disadvantage of an extra operation. Once we learned that avoiding undermining posterior to the maxillary tuberosity would minimize growth disturbance, we began to rely on the straight line von Langenbeck closure of the entire palate, often reinforced by a vomer flap in wider clefts. Palatal lengthening procedures using setback techniques were also performed but had the disadvantage of leaving too much raw surface in the anterior palate. Dr. James Hayward, DDS, head of oral surgery at UM, taught us that extending closure of the soft palatal layers posterior to the uvula (low-draped palate) did in fact functionally lengthen the palate, and we began to use this technique routinely. Finally, recognition of the abnormal anterior orientation of the levator muscle in the cleft encouraged us to reorient the muscle in a horizontal end-on position in the closure of the soft palate. When Furlow's double Z-plasty procedure for closure of the soft palate[97] was reported, we began to use it. We felt it was the operation of choice for submucous clefts but could be problematic on quite wide complete clefts.

In response to the early uncertainty about which cleft closure would produce the best overall long-term result, Dr. Grabb proposed a prospective, randomized long term study.

The project was described in the 1972–73 annual report. A cooperative study of cleft palate surgery would begin in 1970 and was planned to run for at least seven years. Its purpose was to objectively determine which of four different cleft palate repair procedures, selected randomly, would give the best results with regard to speech, facial growth, and hearing.[98] The planning included dentistry, speech, and ENT, in addition to plastic surgery. It was hoped that there would be conclusions within ten years. To acquire the ninety patients[99] needed for the study to have the best chance of statistical significance, Dr. Grabb invited seven other plastic surgery programs from the United States and Canada to participate in the study. To my knowledge, this was one of the nation's first multiinstitutional prospective outcome studies. Unfortunately, when Dr. Grabb died, a lot of the momentum for the study dissipated and the study eventually ebbed before enough patients could have the necessary and required long-term evaluation.

### 4. Cleft Palate Clinics

One of the most important concepts in the management of cleft lip and palate patients was to incorporate a multidisciplinary approach from the very beginning of their care. From the early days of plastic surgery in Ann Arbor, there was general agreement that this was necessary for the best outcome for patients with these deformities after their lip and/or their palates were repaired. Consequently, before the UM section was formed, there was a cleft lip and palate clinic at SJMH. Among the specialties represented, other than plastic surgery, were pediatrics, ENT, speech therapy, and the dental specialties, including pedodontics, orthodontics, and prosthodontics. Dr. Harlan Bloomer of the speech and language department at UM was a long-standing member. Dr. Gene Buatti, DDS, an orthodontist, was also a loyal participant. The children were all seen after the age of five then, at least once a year by all members of the team. This allowed for close coordination in all decisions about care as the child matured. Clinic visits lasted until final treatment procedures were carried out or when the patient reached maturity in the late teenage years. Occasionally, the clinic would see older children or even adults who still needed treatment or were being seen for the first time. After the Section of Plastic Surgery was formed in 1964, the university hospital cleft clinic included, in addition to the specialties listed above, oral surgery, genetics, and pediatric social workers.

### 5. Presurgical Palatal Orthopedics

In treating the UCL alveolar deformity, initially we used a preliminary lip adhesion for the very severe complete cleft. This procedure effectively narrowed the alveolar cleft so as to facilitate the definitive lip repair. However, the scarring from the initial adhesion often made the definitive repair more difficult. We began to use Dr. Pool's suggestion of having the parents, right from the baby's birth, place Steri-Strip tapes on the lip across the cleft in the lead-up to lip repair. We found that this significantly narrowed the alveolar cleft and accomplished almost as much as the lip adhesion did without the additional operation. There were cases, however, where there was significant collapse of the lateral alveolar segment and we needed some way to expand it. Dr. Latham, DDS, had described preoperative maxillary orthopedics as early as 1976.[100] His expansion device was in two pieces, connected by an adjustable plate, and was pinned to the maxillary segments in an operative procedure. The parents gradually expanded the palate by daily turning a small screw. The construction of this device obviously required the collaboration of a pediatric prosthodontist, and one was not always available. The Latham device became most useful in the management of bilateral clefts for controlling the ideal width of the lateral alveolar segments and to help reduce the abnormal forward positioning of the premaxilla. There was general agreement among us that surgical repositioning of the forward projecting premaxilla was detrimental and that it could lead to midface retrusion. We felt getting the lip closed and orbicularis muscle union behind the narrowed prolabium would allow the premaxilla to end up in a more normal position. With wider complete bilateral clefts, bilateral lip adhesions were frequently required, and if there was a very wide cleft and a very protrusive premaxilla, then we would have to stage the adhesions, one side at a time. There was still a fairly high incidence of adhesion dehiscence. One of the ways we found to reduce that possibility was by taking the tension off the closure by a retention suture placed in the muscle through both sides of the lip right under the alar bases. It was an improvement, but we still had a long way to go in the management of the bilateral cleft.

*6. UCL Nose*

Sometime after Harold McComb, from Australia, described his ideas of repositioning the nasal alar cartilage on the cleft side in 1976,[101] and we began to use the technique, our results were encouraging. It was very appealing because, in comparison with other described techniques, it could be accomplished through the existing incisions necessary to repair the lip. As McComb had described, we used two permanent suspension sutures through the upper edge of the cleft-side lateral crus passed subcutaneously and brought out at the nasion and tied over a Steri-Strip. Obviously, this required some subcutaneous dissection from the alar cartilage up over the cartilaginous and bony vault. We discovered it was best to slightly overcorrect the inferiorly displaced alar cartilage. We were pleased with the initial results and gratified when Dr. McComb published his ten-year follow-up in 1985.[102] Correcting the position of the cleft-side alar cartilage completely precluded having to do any nasal tip surgery in the preschool age child. As teenagers, the patients often did need a secondary corrective rhinoplasty to achieve better symmetry in the nose, particularly around the tip, but the remaining deformity was much less severe than in patients who had not had primary nasal repair.

*7. Nasoendoscopy*

In the mid-1970s, when 3-mm flexible fiber optic endoscopes became available, we realized that this would give us the opportunity to directly view the anatomy of palatal closure through the nasopharynx. We had always been able to diagnose velopharyngeal insufficiency by analyzing the patient's speech, and confirm velopharyngeal incompetence by listening to the air leak during speech with a tube placed between the patient's nares and our ear. However, an oral view of the palate in action did not give us the specific information we needed to assess not only the adequacy of closure of the repaired palate but also the specific anatomy of it to assist in planning the advisability of nonsurgical therapy or which type of surgical correction would be necessary. The available radiologic studies required x-ray exposure and did not always give us the desired three-dimensional information we needed. We began to use the endoscope in the outpatient clinic on selected older children. Anesthesia was provided by using topical nasal sprays, and we were impressed with the clarity of palatal function on the video as the patient spoke test words and phrases. Being able to assess the movements of the lateral and posterior pharynx was an added benefit. Endoscopy had become an extremely helpful guide in selecting the procedure likely to be most successful for each of these patients. The results were essential in deciding between the more traditional posterior pharyngeal flap, which was basically static, and the innovative dynamic pharyngoplasty, originally described by Orticochea in 1968[103] and modified by Jackson and Silverton in 1977.[104] Gradually, we were able to study younger children, and many of them enjoyed looking at the recorded videos after the exam. From the beginning, we collaborated with the speech therapists who worked with us in the cleft clinic, and ultimately, they took over doing the exam and were more successful than we were in getting younger children to cooperate. The endoscope was a tremendous advance in the follow-up of all our many cleft palate patients. Drs. Izenberg, Rohrich, VanderKolk, and I published our early experiences in 1985.[105]

*8. Alveolar Bone Grafts*

Over the years, a more collegial relationship developed with the oral surgeons participating in the cleft clinic conferences. We exchanged information freely when we discussed the patients who had been evaluated. One of the benefits of this was that Dr. Ray Fonseca, DDS, head of oral surgery at the time, generously shared with me his technique for closing and bone grafting alveolar clefts in the mixed dentition patient.[106] This involved creating a bed for a cancellous iliac graft by turning in toward the nasal floor the mucosa of the fistula tract, and widely undermining and shifting the palatal tissue to close the nasal side. Undermined maxillary gingival flaps were then shifted toward the midline to close the oral side. This procedure was a big improvement over previous techniques. The iliac bone graft site was rendered much less painful for these children by avoiding any muscle dissection and creating a periosteal-cortical flap for access to the medullary layer that was closed over the extraction site.

## *Rhinoplasty*

Dr. Dingman's openness to new and better ideas led the rest of us to be aware of new advances in rhinoplasty. His friendship with Dr. Joseph Tamerin from New York City led Dr. Tamerin to be visiting professor at UM in 1969. Dr. Tamerin operated on one of our patients with a resident assisting. He used the intracartilaginous (cartilage splitting) incision for approaching the tip in rhinoplasty. This demonstration and the resulting natural-looking tips in the patients that he presented later that day in conference encouraged all of us to start using that approach, moving away from previous experience with either the intercartilaginous retrograde approach or the delivery technique. Then, in 1971, Dr. Dingman sent Carl Berner, resident 1970–72, to an ENT facial plastic surgery rhinoplasty conference, and Carl brought back all sorts of new concepts, including the open approach, that we discussed and began to use with difficult tips, particularly in teaching situations. Carl reported to me recently, "I remember how thrilled I was to be sent by ROD to 'spy' on the facial plastic surgeons regarding their techniques. I had no idea how I would be received, as at that time there was some animosity between the specialties. I need not have been concerned. Dr. Dingman's reputation preceded me. I was welcomed by all. I believe what I learned was valuable to me in my practice and to all of us. Rhinoplasty was a big part of my practice. What I learned through the rhinoplasty meeting gave me more confidence."[107] The friendliness and respect shared by Dr. Dingman and those ENT facial plastic surgeons was in part due to the respect Dr. Dingman had gained by his participating in their teaching conferences and having accepted ENT trainees into our residency program. He once said to me, "There should be no limits on education. You should be willing to teach to whomever wants to learn."[108]

Another "light bulb" experience occurred at an ASPRS meeting in Houston in 1974. Dr. Jack Sheen presented his revolutionary work on the correction of secondary rhinoplasty. We had all been struggling with these deformities. To correct them, we had been removing scar tissue and further reducing dorsal structures to correct the common "pollybeak" deformity. Dr. Sheen turned the tables on us as he showed markedly improved results using augmentation of tip, dorsum, and radix rather than making any further reduction. The underlying concept he presented was to *increase* the structural support and *expand* the skin envelope, thereby improving shape and function. I can remember a collective "gasp" in an audience of about one thousand five hundred plastic surgeons as Dr. Sheen presented what I interpreted as amazingly good results. A better understanding of the underlying concepts of that presentation, published in *PRS* 1975,[109] helped us to define the factors in evaluating a primary rhinoplasty patient that, if uncorrected or made worse, could lead to the necessity for a secondary rhinoplasty. These new concepts helped us to improve the treatment of secondary patients as well as better evaluate our primary rhinoplasty candidates.

Sometime during the early 1980s, I was exposed to the idea of suture techniques to control the shape and position of the tip cartilages. This happened at a university hospital teaching conference in ENT to which I was invited to hear the visiting professor, Dr. Gene Tardy, a well-known facial plastic surgeon. I realized that it was a real advance in rhinoplasty surgery to have available a technique that was very effective, nondestructive, and reversible. Based on this experience, we modified our techniques and significantly improved our results.

Dr. Dingman always placed a high premium on accurate and easily understood terminology to eliminate confusion in discussion of operative details. An example of this attention to detail appeared in the article he and Paul Natvig published in *PRS* in 1982, near the end of both of their careers, clarifying the incisions for rhinoplasty.[110] This article was an effort to clarify by description and illustrations the details and proper names of the incisions used to gain access to the alar cartilages during rhinoplasty. The important distinction between the oft-confused infracartilaginous incision at the caudal edge of the alar cartilage and cephalic to the soft triangle, and more caudal marginal (or rim) incision was graphically illustrated.

In addition to all this stimulating information, the advent of residents coming through the program with prior ENT training gave all the other residents, and particularly those of us on the faculty who were interested in rhinoplasty, an ongoing tutorial on surgery of the nose, especially with regard to the septum and nasal physiology. This group of residents had been schooled in the technique of open rhinoplasty, which had advantages for correcting complicated aesthetic tip deformities, for secondary cases, and especially for cleft lip nasal deformities. As we began to use the open technique, the obvious advantages for OR teaching became evident. One of the most practical suggestions concerning technique came from Erlan Duus (1983–85). He introduced me to a dental instrument, the amalgam tamper, for ease in defining the proper dissection plane in septal surgery. Those old enough to have had dental fillings might remember seeing one. The exact instrument he recommended has small sharp serrations on the square end. I quickly realized that it was very efficient for "scratching" through the perichondrium of the nasal septum down to the proper layer for dissection without cutting into the cartilage. It seemed to me far superior to either scissors or a knife. I found that, after starting the dissection, if I got out of the proper layer, a few "scratches" would put me back into the proper dissection plane.

Dr. Jack Gunter had been acting head of ENT at University of Texas Southwestern (UTSW), prior to starting his plastic surgery residency with us in 1978. Shortly thereafter, he and I recognized our mutual interest in rhinoplasty. He took the time to discuss with me most of my preoperative rhinoplasty cases. He taught me many of the fine points of clinical analysis and operative technique of rhinoplasty that he had learned both from his ENT training and from his fellowship with Dr. Jack Anderson, a well-respected facial plastic surgeon. After he completed the residency at Michigan in 1980 and went back to Dallas, Jack and I talked several times and came up with the idea of a postgraduate course including cadaver dissections, didactic instruction, and patient presentations. We both felt it was necessary to augment plastic surgery rhinoplasty training for residents, and there was also a need for teaching these basic ideas to recent postgraduates. The first course was at UTSW in Dallas in 1982, where Jack was a faculty member. He recruited other faculty from Dallas and Houston, including Sam Stal, Steve Byrd, and John Tebbets. We talked about having a meeting the next year in Ann Arbor and then alternating sites every other year, but Bill Grabb's sudden death put that plan on hold. By the time everything settled down at UM, Dr. Rod Rohrich, another one of our alumni (finished in 1985), had graduated and gone to UTSW to join the faculty. Together with Rod and Jack Gunter, the annual Dallas Rhinoplasty Course became well established there and has continued as one of the premier rhinoplasty international conferences for over thirty years. The formal and informal discussions among the faculty, which included some from ENT, were the stimulus that eventually led to the formation of the Rhinoplasty Society. The nasal anatomy video that Paul Izenberg, Bob Gilman (1980–82), and I created for basic teaching in the Dallas course continues to be useful and a valuable part of the curriculum for teaching our residents rhinoplasty at Michigan.

## Congenital Protruding Ear Deformity

Several events early on contributed to the evolution of our otoplasty technique for protruding ear deformity. Dr. Stenstrom, in 1963, published his technique for shaping the curve of the antihelix with linear abrasions.[111] Dr. Dingman was impressed that this was an excellent idea, and he then developed a new instrument by taking the two halves of a Brown Adson forceps, bending the stems in two different directions and putting a handle on each one so the instrument in the surgeon's hand would easily follow the curve of the antihelix of both the right and left ears. This was the origin of the Dingman ear cartilage abrader, another of ROD's many practical and ingenious modifications. At about the same time, Mr. John Mustarde of Scotland, later to honor UM as visiting professor, described the use of mattress sutures to create a gently curved antihelix.[112] In younger children with more pliable cartilage, probably with either the abrasion or the mattress sutures, the correction would hold up over the long term. However, we felt that it was safer to create the curve by abrasion and then use the mattress sutures for more secure reinforcement. This combination of techniques seemed to be particularly useful in older children or adult patients where more mature, stiffer cartilage might cause the deformity to reoccur after either simple abrasion or just the mattress sutures. Later, in 1979, Dr. Isaac Peled, one of our fellows from Israel, and Dr. Dingman described a modified technique.[113] The final important key to success in our otoplasty evolution was provided by Dr. David Furnas in 1978 whose published article demonstrated that reducing the overprojecting posterior concha wall did not require cartilage excision but it could be repositioned posteriorly with the use of concha-mastoid sutures.[114] The repositioning of the concha was aided by slightly thinning the floor of the concha and removing adjacent soft tissue just posterior to it, thus leaving a space in which the concha could be set back. Another technical aspect was realizing that the standard elliptical postauricular excision when closed could overcorrect the frontal profile of the middle of the external ear. We found that a dumbbell-shaped incision was more desirable and much less likely to cause overcorrection. Otoplasty for protruding ears was one of the most satisfying operations for the patient and surgeon. It was a delight to observe the excited positive response when patients, both young and old, viewed themselves in a mirror at the time of dressing removal.

## Face-Lift Experience

The procedure of face-lifting early on was basically a subcutaneous dissection and tightening of the skin, frequently associated with bilateral upper and lower lid blepharoplasty. All this began to change after the publication of Dr. Tord Skoog's book in 1974 about the deep fascial dissection in the face.[115] Then, in 1976, Drs. Mitz and Peyronie published a detailed description of the SMAS (subcutaneous musculo-aponeurotic system) fascial layer in the face.[116] Because of the improvement in the nasolabial fold and less tension on the dissected skin cheek flaps, there was subsequently a lot of enthusiasm for using these newer deeper dissections. Moreover, coming into common usage were procedures on the platysma muscle, in which the lateral portion of the muscle is divided and then suspended, thereby tightening the still-undissected overlying skin. We also realized that a submental Z-plasty of the central platysmal bands could improve the anterior neck contour. This was associated with procedures of imbricating the subdermal soft tissues under the chin to correct the "witch's chin" look. We also used selective chin augmentation to improve the acuteness of the cervical-mental angle. In 1985, after the introduction of cannulas for liposuction, we began to use small, flat, blunt cannulas as subcutaneous dissectors for the cheek and neck. This idea was introduced to me by one of our residents, Abram Nguyen (resident, 1985–87). This technique proved to be less traumatic than sharp dissection. We found that with gentle pressure, we could create subcutaneous tunnels in the proper plane that could later be connected by selective sharp dissection under direct vision.

The deep plane dissection techniques continued to evolve but those of us favoring a more conservative approach began to rely on plication of the SMAS layer and then began to use the lateral SMASectomy described at a meeting by Daniel Baker of New York City.[117] We were influenced by the article by Baker and Conley in 1979 about danger of facial nerve injuries during face-lifts.[118] It certainly encouraged us to take a more critical look at the deep plane approaches because of the possible injuries to branches of the facial nerve. Conley and Baker very clearly outlined the anatomy of the various branches of the nerve and how they might be damaged by some of the techniques in use at the time. The article described in detail the course of the ramus mandibularis of seventh nerve and showed it to be much more variable in its relation to the lower border of the mandible than the description in the study of preserved cadavers by Dingman and Grabb in 1961. This supported our conviction that it was essential to use fresh cadaver material for all our anatomic dissections for them to be reliably translated into clinical situations. We followed that in subsequent anatomic dissection projects. We also paid close attention to Peter McKenny's description in 1980 of how to avoid injury to the greater auricular nerve in the posterior neck.[119]

In 1977, Dr. Ron Wexler published an article concerning possible incisions for male face-lifts based on the experience he gained while at Jackson Prison as a resident.[120] He emphasized the importance of and illustrated techniques to ensure leaving adequate hairless preauricular skin posterior to the sideburn at the end of the procedure.

Paul Dempsey (resident, 1976–78), who finished his training along with Eric Austad and Paul Izenberg, introduced to us in the early 1980s the concept of a subperiosteal approach through a coronal incision to elevate the midface. Dr. Izenberg and I did fresh cadaver dissections to help define the fascial relationships in the lateral forehead and dissection down to the zygomatic arch where a subperiosteal dissection over the zygoma allowed safe dissection and suspension of the deeper layers of the midface.

During those years, we became convinced that it was very important to determine whether the aging patient's preoperative rationale for improvement was based on her own feelings of decreased self-esteem, or on wishing to have career advancement with a more youthful appearance. We found that these valid patient desires correlated well with the best assurance of a satisfied and happy patient postoperatively. This kind of preoperative assessment required a thorough pre-op interview using a lot of open-ended questions to ensure that the patient's motivation was not based on something her husband or a friend might be insisting on. The value of this approach was confirmed by a study by Goin, Burgoyne, and Goin in 1980. They reported that a patient's desire to "improve their self-image and to advance their career were reasonably reliable predictors of [postoperative] psychological improvement."[121] In addition, we were always concerned about the effect of smoking in face-lift patients and usually required them to stop smoking for at least six weeks preoperatively. Our concern was confirmed by a study reported by Rees in 1984 that smoking did increase the risk for cheek flap vascular impairment postoperatively.[122] We also applied this rationale to operations such as abdominoplasty and even, in some cases, reduction mammoplasty and breast ptosis.

## Brow-Lift and Blepharoplasty

Drs. Dingman, Peled, and Izenberg stated at the beginning of their article in 1979, "Forehead wrinkles, drooping eyebrows, and blepharoptosis are some of the earliest signs of the aging face. Loss of skin elasticity in conjunction with gravitational forces upon the forehead, brow, and upper lids results in a constant tired or angry expression. These changes are progressive . . . and do not reflect the patient's true personality. Attempts to correct this condition by [eyelid] skin excision alone are usually ineffective and disappointing to both patient and surgeon."[123]

This point of view reflected very accurately the importance that Dr. Dingman always stressed, with both the faculty and residents, of assessing the whole face whenever evaluating a patient's aging changes. Seeing post-op patients with him in his office, we were witness to the profoundly positive effect that the alleviation of the "tired and angry" look had for the patient, often as, or more, important than improvement in the lower face. The article also discussed the various approaches for these corrections, including transcoronal, either through the scalp or at the hairline in cases of high foreheads in females or also under special circumstances, that is, a male patient, using a forehead wrinkle for access. These approaches were all eventually superseded by the endoscopic approach to forehead and brow-lifts.

We were all influenced by the seminal work presented by Dr. Salvador Castanares describing the anatomy of the herniated intraorbital fat and how to deal with it safely during blepharoplasty surgery. His work became the mainstay of our approach to "baggy eyelids."[124] During those years, we were also constantly reevaluating our results with blepharoplasty. We gradually became more conservative about fat removal in the upper lids, except for the nasal fat compartment, in an effort to avoid the "hollowed out" look. We also removed less upper eyelid skin in conjunction with brow-lifts, thereby minimizing the risk of a post-op patient being unable to close his or her upper lids comfortably, especially at night. In the lower lids, we always had the patient (under local and light sedation) open his or her mouth widely before excising the lower lid skin. Using skin-muscle flaps and tightening the orbicularis laterally helped. These were the days before common use of canthopexy. We also repaired senile ptosis due to levator dehiscence, but routinely referred the congenital cases to pediatric ophthalmology. When patients presented as adults with an unclear history, a high school photograph was most helpful in ruling out whether the ptosis might be congenital. We were also on the lookout for cases of myasthenia gravis that can sometimes present with ptosis as an initial symptom to avoid surgery and make sure the patient received proper medical evaluation and treatment.

Mr. John Mustarde of Scotland was a good friend of Dr. Dingman's and a visiting professor more than once, as well as a fishing companion. He graciously introduced all of us to the fundamental principles of reconstruction of resected and traumatized eyelids. His famous book *Repair and Reconstruction in the Orbital Region*[125] became a bible for us and provided a basis for dealing with many complex problems. We all felt deeply indebted to this very learned and charming Scotsman (Photo 56).

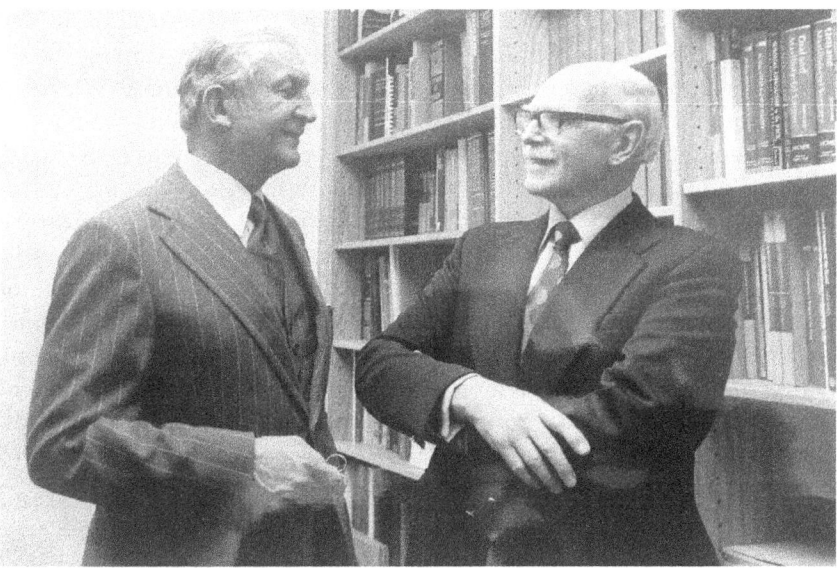

Photo 56: Mr. John Mustarde, visiting professor from Scotland, with Dr. Dingman in the Dingman Library.

## Liposuction

Although the use of suction and a sharp curette to remove subcutaneous fat was first published in *PRS* in 1978,[126] this idea did not receive much attention until, in 1983, Dr. Illouz of France published his results of lipolysis in three thousand cases, having performed it since 1977.[127] There was a lot of skepticism about the technique in the United States, but finally the ASPRS appointed a committee to evaluate the procedure. A group of plastic surgeons went over to France and came back with rather glowing reports after spending time with Dr. Illouz and evaluating his work. There were arguments whether the technique should be wet or dry, but the wet technique of Dr. Illouz seemed to have less bleeding associated with it.

There were some postgraduate teaching conferences on liposuction set up by respected plastic surgeons, and several of our faculty and residents attended these training sessions. Many of us became convinced that the technique, as described by Dr. Illouz, was effective with minimal morbidity in the removal of localized collections of unaesthetic subcutaneous fat accumulation. It seemed to be particularly useful in the lateral hips, abdomen, and in the submental area of the neck. We were also sure that this was not indicated as a substitute method of weight loss in truly obese patients.

The worry about overcorrection was frequently an issue with the then available large diameter cannulas. As small diameter blunt cannulas became available, they allowed much more finesse in removal of fat and avoided getting too superficial where it might result in rippling under the skin, one of the complications of this type of procedure. When the tumescent technique of infiltrating large volumes of saline containing very dilute local anesthesia and very dilute epinephrine was introduced, it became possible to carry out the procedure in an ambulatory setting with supplemental IV sedation. With greater experience, we learned some of the limitations of this procedure early on and tended to avoid the medial thighs, because the skin did not contract well. We had some good results, and ultimately, we were able to combine lateral flank liposuction together with the standard abdominoplasty, but avoiding suction in the abdominal flap. It is interesting to note that currently some type of liposuction is the most common aesthetic operation performed in this country. Of course, liposuction has gone on to much wider use, including collecting fat for autogenous fat transplantation.

## *Facial Fractures*

With the publication of their book, *Surgery of Facial Fractures*, in 1964,[128] Drs. Dingman and Natvig brought the fundamentals of caring for these injuries to our attention in Ann Arbor, as well as to the plastic surgery community and the world beyond. It bears mention that Dr. Child, whose political skills supported the development and formation of the Section of Plastic Surgery in the years leading up to the publication, wrote the foreword to the book. It is only speculation, but one wonders if the high regard for the authors expressed in the foreword reflected his expectation of Dr. Dingman's potential as a great teacher. Quoting Dr. Child, "The text by Doctors Dingman and Natvig encompasses past and present knowledge of facial fractures. It clearly points the way toward a better understanding of one of surgery's most humanitarian accomplishments: the mending of fractured faces . . . the authors . . . have captured the past with charm and the present with vigor. The ability to teach their skills by word and by picture is limited only by their student's capacity and motivation to learn."[129]

The book's publication preceded by two years President Lyndon Johnson's signing the law making automobile seat belts mandatory in 1968. However, it was not until the mid-1970s, when the development of the enhanced seatbelt reminder (ESBR) became universal and seatbelt usage increased from around 15 percent to 70 percent, that these serious facial injuries saw a marked reduction. So for the first ten years after publication, all types of facial fractures were always a big part of our practice. Dingman and Natvig's book provided a description of types of injuries for each anatomic location as well as step-by-step illustrations of the necessary corrective maneuvers, and the book became an essential guide for surgical correction. The authors described and illustrated the use of the internal suspension sutures from a stable frontal bone to facilitate intraoral suspension of the maxilla so necessary in the management of those complex cases of skull-facial bone disjunction. The epilogue of the book was written by G. Kasten Tallmadge, a colleague of Dr. Natvig's at Marquette Medical School and a friend of Dr. Dingman's. It is a beautiful description of the part of the body so intrinsic to the art of plastic surgery. Quoting in part, "Is there another part of the body which is more nearly one's self than the face? The incredibly complex arrangements of the parts from the microscopic to the massive have given to man alone . . . the power of intelligible speech and the great gift of his ability to make music. The ceaselessly mobile lines of the countenance conceal or reveal the recondite workings of the spirit."[130]

Although car safety improvements significantly reduced their incidence, facial fractures resulting from a variety of other etiologies remained a significant part of our trauma care. As an aside, I learned the hard way about the importance of knowledge of pre-op occlusion in conjunction with a case of a patient with LeFort II midface fractures along with mandible fracture. At operation, we applied the direct interosseous wiring and suspension wiring techniques. I got the displaced structures back into what I thought was very nice occlusion. By the next morning, the patient had pushed his lower jaw forward and was in a Class III relationship. I was confused by it but his mother said, "You know I think he may have always looked like that." Because the patient lived locally, we contacted his dentist and obtained his pre-op dental impressions and realized that he was prognathic before the injury. It was a good lesson to me to always know as much as you can about a patient preoperatively.

*Naso-orbital fractures* were one specific type of severe facial fractures not discussed in great detail in Drs. Dingman and Natvig's book. Early on, we recognized the uniqueness of these complex injuries from a frontal force pushing the nasal mass posteriorly into the lacrimal-ethmoid structures. Associated fractures of the frontal sinus often involved the posterior wall and the anterior cranial fossa. To achieve an accurate diagnosis, the clinical exam and regular x-rays had to be followed by open reduction. Direct wire fixation was necessary after reducing all the displaced fragments, along with both neurosurgical and ENT consultation for management of the frontal sinus fractures unless the injury was restricted to the anterior wall of the sinus. By 1969, Drs. Dingman, Grabb, and I had gained enough experience with these cases to report our findings in *Archives of Surgery*.[131] In 1979, Drs. Dingman and Izenberg contributed a comprehensive review of the possible complications of facial fractures as well as facial soft tissue injuries in John Conley's textbook on head and neck surgery complications.[132]

## Maxillofacial Surgery

This was a special interest of Dr. Dingman's from the beginning of his career. We were all intrigued by the collaboration that had developed between him and an inventive orthodontist in Ann Arbor, Dr. Robert Ponitz, DDS (Photo 57). Once a decision was made as to whether the maxilla, mandible, or both were to be modified, Dr. Ponitz made models and splints to show exactly what had to be done and what the exact dental occlusion was to be postoperatively. He excelled in doing preoperative orthodontics so that when the surgery was done, the teeth fit nicely together in the most desirable occlusal relationship. This collaboration had led to the evolution of quite sophisticated planning and immobilization techniques. For those of us who were not trained in dentistry and the fundamentals of dental occlusion, it was a bit of an uphill battle to learn these concepts, but by working closely with Dr. Dingman, we were encouraged to branch out on our own with the help of his close friend and colleague, Dr. Ponitz. Many of our maxillofacial patients were adults with secondary cleft lip sequelae who had orthognathic deformities. Before the sagittal split mandibular procedure achieved popularity (it was never favored by either ROD or Dr. Ponitz), we performed vertical ramus osteotomies or body ostectomies for mandibular setback. We would often go to Dr. Ponitz's office before the case and go over the cephalograms and the models, and look at the splints. He was extremely cooperative and so interested in the actual surgery that he would join us in the OR. As he was a member of the medical staff at SJMH, he could scrub in and assist us, and his on-the-spot analysis was always helpful.

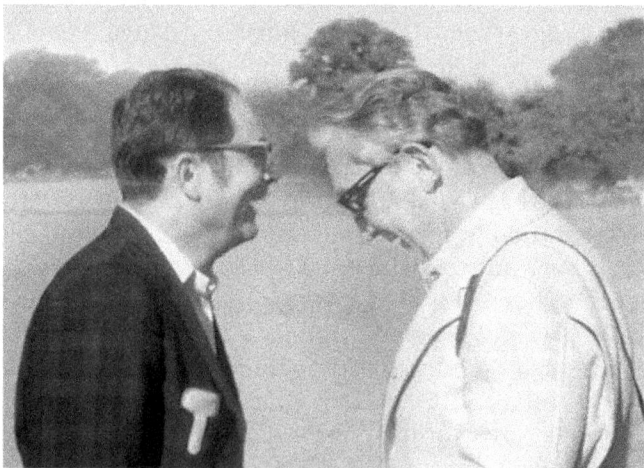

Photo 57: Robert Ponitz, DDS, speaking with Dr. Dingman at a Grabb balloon launching.

An interesting example of this collaboration with Dr. Ponitz to solve a unique clinical problem was published in 1969 in *PRS*.[133] The article referred to a previous successful case (from another institution) of functional sternocleidomastoid muscle (SCM) transfer to treat masseter muscle atrophy secondary to poliomyelitis. The patient in the current article had congenital absence of bilateral masseter muscles. Seen as a teenager, he was unable to actively close his mouth, having to position his chin on his chest and push his head forward to achieve closure. He also had a massive open-bite deformity and absence of mandibular angles. Two mandibular body osteotomies and iliac bone grafts were required to reshape the mandible. Both SCM muscles were transferred on pedicles containing the accessory nerve and occipital artery. They were positioned between the zygoma and lower border of the mandible. Both transferred muscles regained their function and allowed the patient to actively close his mouth. Dr. Hudak related to me his experience with another application of transferring the SCM:

> Looking back, I had the opportunity as a resident to do a facial reconstruction using the sternocleidomastoid muscle for facial atrophy. That procedure done in 1969 was a forerunner of many of those procedures that followed using muscle for breast reconstruction as well as free muscle grafts. I wrote a paper on the case: Sternocleidomastoid Flap for Correction of Soft Tissue Defects of the Face which I presented at the National Residents Conference in Salt Lake City in 1970. I won the award for the Outstanding Paper for Head and Neck Reconstruction. I think this was one of the first muscle trans-positioning papers.[134]

Dr. Dingman, over the years, attracted many patients who were suffering from malfunction of the TMJs from a variety of causes. Many of them were severely symptomatic. He worked out a safe surgical approach to both the upper and lower aspects of the joint, allowing him to refine his surgical procedures. He reported his surgical results in two articles: the first with 440 cases in 1969 coauthored with a resident at the time, Dr. Eric Constant,[135] and the second in 1975, coauthored with another resident, Dr. Richard Lawrence and Dr. Dingman's son David, a plastic surgeon on the faculty of the University of Utah, reporting on another twenty-five cases.[136] The surgical approach to the TMJ was thoroughly described and illustrated. A significant proportion of the patients benefited from the variety of surgical procedures.

During these years and subsequently, it was discovered that one of the main underlying etiologic factors leading to dysfunction of the TMJ was unresolved traumatic dental occlusion. Recognition and correction of it as well as prevention of the resulting chronic stress on the TMJ, with a removable dental splint worn at night, ultimately resulted in a significant diminution of the difficult cases. After being contacted by the authors for comment about the TMJ reports, Dave Dingman replied,

> It is a hard subject to discuss. The real cases such as the originals and some of mine had real pathology. I chased many of these cases down by flying around the country and the results were dramatic, with normal pain free function decades after the surgery. One such case was a girl from Honduras that had bilateral ankyloses. It was a big deal in the local papers as it was an Interplast case and the child stayed a while and became friends with my twins. She did not want to leave. Some of the bad results were patients who had prosthetic joint implants. Some got infected and the results were not good. I am not sure about the role good dentistry played [in prevention of TMJ dysfunction] but I am sure it was a factor. Some of the reduction in the number of surgical cases may have been due to alleviation of the secondary TMJ symptoms in depressed patients when treated with new and better anti-depressant medication.[137]

Dr. Dingman also did a lot of other types of maxillary surgery, and there were always the possibility of risks. Dr. Lenny Glass (1968–70) recounted such a tragic case during his time as a resident, "I remember so vividly the teenager who exsanguinated in his hospital bed apparently from iatrogenic damage to his carotid artery (a rare complication) which occurred five to six days previously during one of ROD's first LeFort II advancements. I never forgot that. A curved osteotome was used to blindly separate the perpendicular plate from the maxilla. Seemed too risky a procedure to do without visualization so I never did one.[138] It is probably important to emphasize the dangers and risks faced by pioneers like Dr. Dingman in performing these difficult procedures for the first time. We do not always remember the debt we owe to these innovators as these complex operations can now be performed much more safely on a routine basis.

Another recollection came from Bruce Novark (1972–74) about ROD's open-mindedness in regard to residents' assessments of a problem:

> As renowned an icon as he was, he would always listen to our input and critiques. We saw a 26-year-old woman in clinic with an apparent prominent mandible and class III malocclusion. The chief thought she needed mandibular surgery, I wasn't so sure. Further clinical exam and cephalometric analysis demonstrated the problem to be in the midface. I presented my evidence and belief that she needed a LeFort II naso-maxillary advancement. (Don't think one had been done at the U of M at that time.) The boss listened, agreed (he didn't say, "no we'll do it my way"), and I went ahead with the procedure with his assistance. ROD was that kind of guy.[139]

## Lip Reconstruction

Dr. Dingman demonstrated his characteristic interest in innovation in two instances with ideas suggested by residents. One was with Ron Wexler (1970–72) in reporting a case of a large subtotal excision of the lower lip excluding the commissures in an older patient with a redundant upper lip. The article described two Stein-Eslander Abbe style flaps that were designed to extend up just lateral to the nose and rotated into the lower lip on skeletonized superior labial arterial pedicles. These were divided in a couple of weeks providing adequate functioning lip balance in a difficult situation.[140] The other instance was with Grant Fairbanks (1969–71), who thus described it:

> Dr. Dingman was always interested in publishing new techniques if he thought it could benefit the patients and the profession. On one occasion, I was recreating the oral commissure on a woman who had lost this portion of her lip in an auto accident. Dr. Dingman came in and looked over our shoulders and asked me what I was doing. I explained the approach and stated that I had performed a similar procedure while serving on the Hospital Ship Hope in Tunis which Dr. Dingman had arranged for me through his friend at Sinai Hospital in Detroit, Herbert Bloom, DDS. He told me this was a new procedure and it should be presented.[141] (It was presented at ASPRS 1971 and published in *PRS* in 1972.[142])

## Introduction of Craniofacial Surgery to Michigan

Dr. Haskell Newman related in detail the sequence of events that brought craniofacial surgery to Michigan and its subsequent developments:

> In 1967, Dr. Paul Tessier presented the first successful case in which a facial advancement was performed to treat a patient with Crouzon Syndrome. A publication described the technique.[143] A Le Fort III osteotomy advancement was designed to include a major portion of the orbits with the upper jaw. This technique of dissecting tissue from the facial bones with simultaneous intracranial exposure and circumferential mobilization of the orbits enabled repositioning of the eyes and the skull. Tessier's techniques are based on the principle that skull and facial bones must be repositioned or reconstructed before soft tissue can be repaired. In the early 1970s, surgeons from the United States visited Tessier to learn the new operative techniques. Among his early students was Reed Dingman, Chairman of the Section of Plastic Surgery at the University of Michigan.[144]

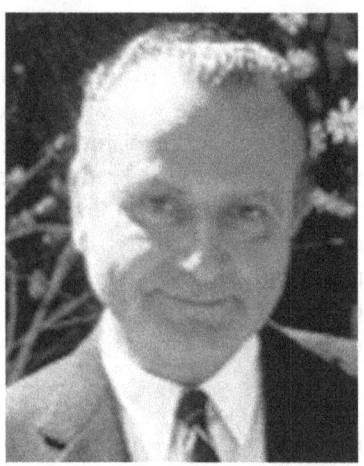

Photo 58: John M. Converse, MD.

Dr. Glass (1970–71) also recalled that "as soon as Paul Tessier (from France) told the world about his work, ROD had the guts, interest, and stamina to embrace this new discipline called craniofacial surgery and started doing cases."[145] Dr. Newman continued, "In 1970, Dr Dingman initiated craniofacial surgery at the university when he accomplished the surgical correction of a patient with Crouzon craniofacial deformity assisted by a university neurosurgeon and Dr. John Converse, the chairman of plastic surgery, New York University"[146] (Photo 58). This event was remembered by Dr. Hudak who recounted, "One of our most interesting visiting professors was John Converse. We had the opportunity to see him and Dr. Dingman operate on a child with Crouzon Syndrome. That was a unique experience for all who witnessed the operation. It took place in the year 1969–70, which was my second year as resident."[147] Dr. Wexler recollected a subsequent case that took place in 1972.[148]

Dr. Newman recalled,

> In the fall of that year, I was an assistant professor in the Department of Otolaryngology and I applied for a residency position in plastic surgery. The interview with Dr. Dingman centered on a joint interest in the developing specialty of craniofacial surgery. After completing the residency in plastic surgery, encouraged by Drs. Dingman and Grabb, I completed a fellowship of craniofacial surgery with Dr. Ian Munro at the University of Toronto, and in 1978, I was recruited by Dr. Grabb to establish a multidisciplinary team to provide consistency and safety with the most advanced treatment for patients suffering from craniofacial anomalies.
>
> The plastic surgery faculty with interest and training in the correction of craniofacial anomalies was expanded in 1981 with the addition of Dr. Lou Argenta following his fellowship training with Dr. Tessier in Paris [Photo 59]. In 1982, Dr. Newman confined his practice to SJMH and Dr. Argenta directed the craniofacial program at the University of Michigan Hospital systems until his departure in 1988. Adult craniofacial and maxillofacial surgery and specialty training were expanded in practices at the university hospital and SJMH. Neurosurgical participation in the

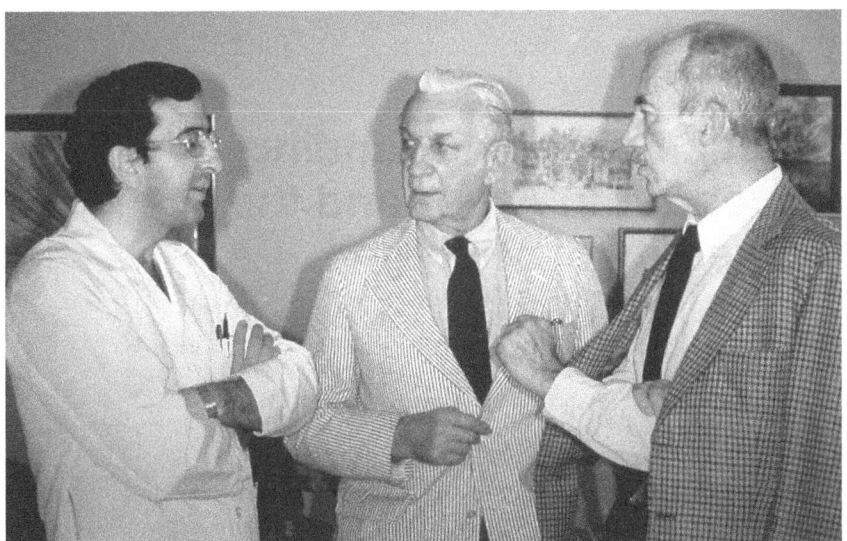

Photo 59: Drs. Argenta, Dingman, and Tessier.

craniofacial program was enhanced when, in 1983, Dr. Joan Venes was recruited to establish and head a division of pediatric neurosurgery. Through the combined interest and efforts of Dr. Venes and the plastic surgery faculty, craniofacial surgical focus expanded to include early interventional correction of craniofacial deformities in infants and young children.[149]

CHAPTER EIGHT

# Plastic Surgery Extending Beyond Ann Arbor and the University of Michigan

We now move on to document the development and growth of the University of Michigan (UM) plastic surgery alumni organization, the Reed O. Dingman (ROD) Society. In addition, we trace the history and development of the Michigan Academy of Plastic Surgery (MAPS), our state plastic surgery society, that was initiated by Dr. Dingman and has contributed greatly to the education and collegiality of the plastic surgeons of Michigan and surrounding states.

## Evolution of the Reed O. Dingman Society

At the 1963 meeting of the American Society of Plastic and Reconstructive Surgery (ASPRS) in Washington, D.C., there was a gathering of preceptees and residents who had trained in the plastic surgery training program at Saint Joseph Mercy Hospital (SJMH) in the previous fifteen years. Their purpose was to form the Reed O. Dingman Society to honor Dr. Dingman by recognizing his excellence as a teacher, his skill as a surgeon, and his greatness as a man. The original diploma presented to him that evening stated that the "aim of the Society was to perfect the art of plastic surgery by sharing knowledge among its colleagues" (see Photo 60). It was signed and dated by the following trainees:

| Clyde Litton | 1948–50 | William C. Grabb | 1959–61 |
|---|---|---|---|
| Wilmer C. Hansen | 1950–52 | Cesar Lozoya Olivas | 1962 |
| Leon Hernandez | 1953–55 | J. Gordon Bell | 1960–61 |
| Paul Natvig | 1955–57 | James R. Stilwell | 1960–62 |
| Merritt C. Mauzy | 1957–59 | Otto Yum-Tu Au | 1961–63 |
| John R. Alger | 1958–60 | Joseph I. Fox | 1963 |
| G. M. Narayanaswamy | 1959–60 | Morgan L. Lucid | 1962–63 |

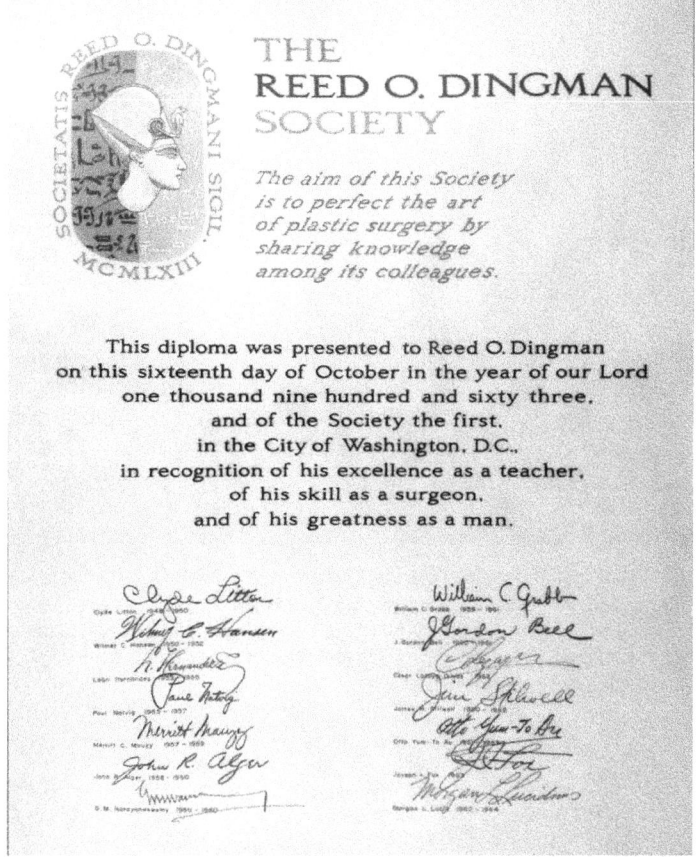

Photo 60: The plaque, motto, and signers initiating the ROD Society.

A photograph was taken of the new society's members at that first meeting (see Photo 61). For the next several years, there was an annual gathering of the society members, either a cocktail party or a dinner that was held at the time and place of the annual meeting of ASPRS. Official photographs of the members and guests were also taken at these subsequent meetings (see Photo 62).

Sometime around 1980, Dr. Dingman returned from attending a meeting of the Ralph Millard Society. He reported enthusiastically that the meeting was a well-attended scientific session apart from being a social gathering. In discussions with him, we got the distinct impression that he felt it was time to add a scientific program to the ROD Society's annual meeting. Subsequently, Dr. Dingman sent a letter to Dr. Grabb who appointed a committee to discuss changing the format of the society to include scientific sessions (see Appendix A-9, p. 158–9,

122  *Plastic Surgery Extending Beyond Ann Arbor*

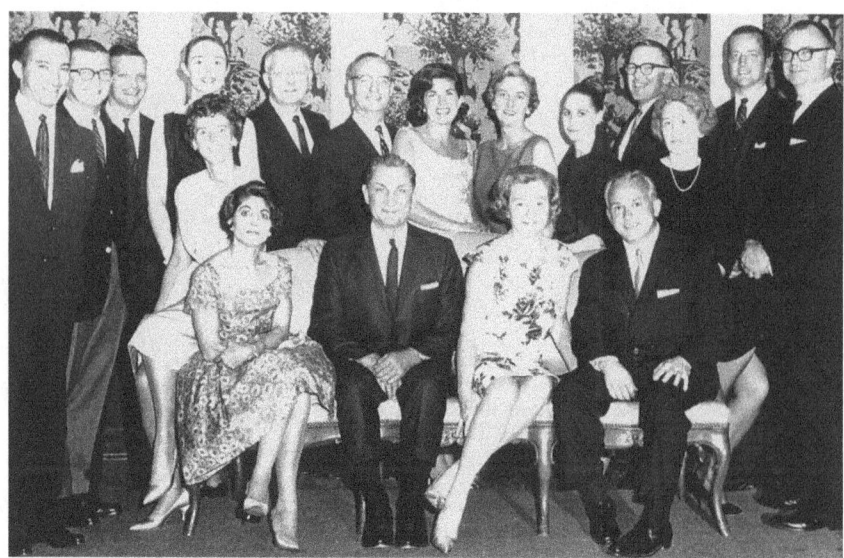

*Photo 61:* Members and guests at the meeting where the Reed O. Dingman Society was formed: from left to right—front: Sophie Hernandez, Reed Dingman, Thelma Dingman, Wilmer Hansen; sitting: Lois Stilwell, Dolly Mauzy; standing: Leon Hernandez, Jim Stilwell, Jack Alger, Ann Natvig, Paul Natvig, Gordon Bell, Cozy Grabb, June Lucid, Mrs. Bell, Morgan Lucid, Bill Grabb, Merritt Mauzy.

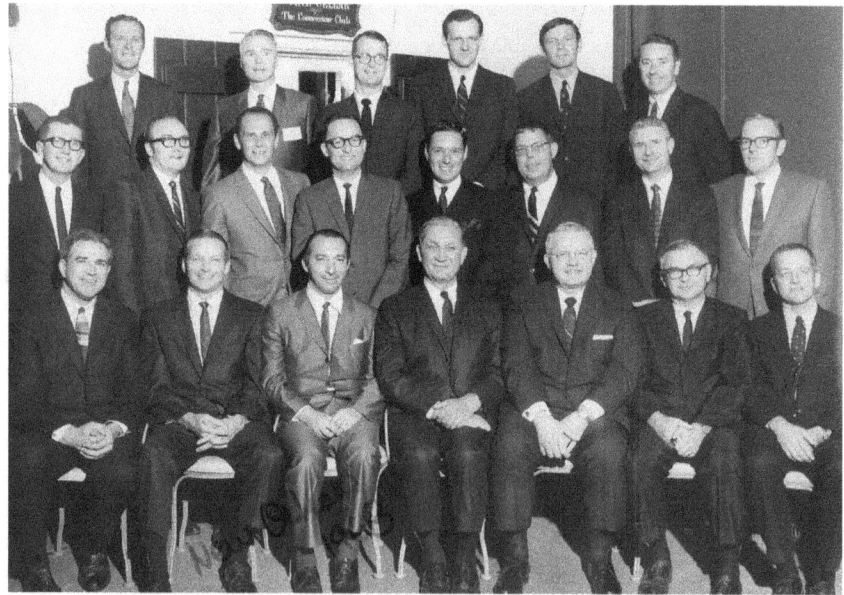

*Photo 62:* Members at the annual meeting of the ROD Society 1968: sitting: No ID, Jack Alger, Leon Hernandez, Reed Dingman, Paul Natvig, Merritt Mauzy, Bill Grabb; first row: Jim Stilwell, John Tipton, Bob Knode, Steve Borocz, Harvey Weiss, Joe Fox, Jim Russell, Morgan Lucid; second row: Fred Speirs, Earl Norling, Don Davis, Ralph Seaton, Ted Dodenhoff, Lenny Glass.

for letters from Drs. Dingman and Grabb). Over the next year or so, Drs. Glass, Berner, Fairbanks, Markley, Izenberg, and I wrote the current bylaws, formalizing the society and reorganizing the format for yearly meetings to include a scientific program. Another objective was to set the precedent that the society was to become the official alumni society of the now thriving UM plastic surgery residency program. We also discussed ways to enlarge membership by extending eligibility to residents who trained in a plastic surgery residency program with a previous UM faculty member or with a resident alumnus on the faculty. Our objective was to have the first meeting under the new format while Dr. Dingman could attend, and this was accomplished. Thus, the first meeting was held in Ann Arbor in 1980. Dr. Dingman made it clear that he approved and appreciated the changes in the format and direction of the society. (Two letters in the appendix [A-9] provide more details of the genesis of the transformation of the society from social to scientific.) After Dr. Grabb's death in 1982, the William Grabb Lectureship was established by the Reed O. Dingman Society through a generous gift from Mrs. Cozette Grabb in memory of her husband. The lectureship was to sponsor a distinguished lecturer to speak at each subsequent society meeting.

Dr. Dingman died in December 1985. Dr. Grant Fairbanks recalled a memorial for Dr. Dingman that the society held in Ann Arbor in June 1986. Quoting Dr. Fairbanks,

> We held a brief memorial for Dr. Dingman at the Dingman Society meeting in the Towsley Center during the summer of 1986. The bronze portrait bust of Reed O. Dingman, sculpted by my father, Avard T. Fairbanks, would stand in for Reed's absence. After a seemingly endless moment of silence and with sadness, we resumed the scientific program. It would be up to all of us to continue the professional legacy he had begun. We are the product of his many years of tireless and selfless service and training. Our patients and those doctors whom we in turn train are the benefactors of the legacy begun by the eminent professor of surgery, Reed O. Dingman, MD, who with foresight, courage, and tireless effort developed the Plastic Surgery Program at the University of Michigan. The program he started has continued in a position of preeminence among plastic surgery training programs as he would have had it [see Photo 63].[1]

The ROD Society has remained very active through the years and continues to function as the official alumni organization of the UM plastic surgery training program.

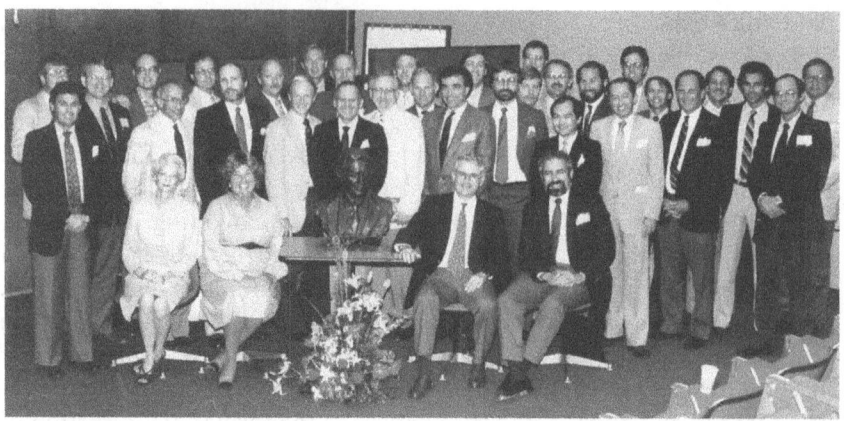

*Photo 63:* Group photograph of the ROD Society members at the memorial for Dr. Dingman in June 1986.

## History of the MAPS

Quoting Dr. Dingman,

> In the early 1950s, I spoke with Bill Lange, Ralph Blocksma, and Wally Steffensen about the advisability of organizing the Michigan plastic surgeons for both scientific and political reasons. In the fall of 1955, we met for lunch in the Founder's Room at the Michigan Union in Ann Arbor and developed organizational plans for a forum to discuss problems in plastic surgery. Then, by letter, I invited all the plastic surgeons in Michigan who were diplomates of the American Board of Plastic Surgery to come to Ann Arbor for a meeting. The meeting was held on June 16, 1956, in a small dining room at the University of Michigan Union. Attending this initial meeting were Drs. Hardy Bethea, Ralph Blocksma, Robert Clifford, Robert J. Meade, William Lange, Wallace Steffansen, and myself. At the first meeting, we decided to meet informally at least once a year to discuss mutual problems, but not get involved in another Society. Chief concerns were third-party insurance carriers, especially the growing and ever-increasing Blue Cross/Blue Shield organizations. The group met at yearly intervals for the first two or three years, and finally it was decided that there should be a constitution and bylaws to assess dues and have more frequent and regular meetings for scientific, legal, and tax reasons. I was elected as the first president of the academy in 1958 and held office until 1960 when Dr. William Lange became the second president.
>
> By 1962, the academy had grown to thirteen full voting members who were board certified and thirteen candidate members who had

completed their training but had not yet qualified by examination. The academy continued to grow in numbers and in importance throughout the State of Michigan. Its sphere of influence became statewide and stronger as new younger men entered the field of plastic surgery and settled in Kalamazoo, Battle Creek, Pontiac, Flint, Saginaw, Muskegon, Oak Park, Southfield, and Grosse Pointe. About 1965, a Section in Plastic Surgery was reorganized by the Michigan State Medical Society, and the academy was asked to name a leading plastic surgeon to conduct special sessions for plastic surgery during the course of the Annual State Medical Society Meetings. Legal and insurance issues became more numerous and the academy began to have meetings at more frequent intervals. In 1965, the bylaws were changed to require four regular scheduled meetings each year. Although a lively interest in economics, medical politics, and malpractice insurance continued to motivate our membership, the meetings progressively became important forums for the discussion of plastic surgery problems with more scientific presentations. The first of the vacation/summer meetings was held on Mackinac Island in July 1968 and the second in July 1970. It was then decided to have the summer meetings at intervals of two years.[2]

Scientific presentations by members and invited guests have improved the content and quality of these meetings. MAPS has become a very important forum for residents from all training programs of the State of Michigan to present their research to a critical audience and get constructive feedback. The casual fellowship has been a valuable way to renew old friendships and initiate new ones. The Mackinac meeting of the academy has also become increasingly popular for doctors and their families from several adjacent states who have joined with us Michiganders to make this meeting a very productive forum for friendship and exchange of scientific thought and new ideas.

CHAPTER NINE

# Reflections and Commentary about Their Ann Arbor Plastic Surgery Experience by the Authors, Residents, and Fellows

All the alumni, residents, and fellows were asked to comment on their memories of the residency training program during the Dingman-Grabb era. Their comments follow, both quoted and, with permission, edited.

Ernie Manders wrote,

> Harken back with me to a golden era in the history of plastic and reconstructive surgery. It was a time of schooling up for the intellectual land rush that was to become modern plastic surgery. Drs. Reed O. Dingman and William C. Grabb had established a Division of Plastic Surgery at the University of Michigan. At last, our specialty had a place at the academic table. Despite the vision of these two leaders, were they standing here today, I have no doubt that both would be immensely surprised—and gratified, at the view of plastic and reconstructive surgery today.
>
> Were our founders here, they would be most happy to see the enduring friendships and loyalties that they and their staff inspired. They would be amazed at the development and everyday use of muscle flaps, free flaps, tissue expansion, breast reconstruction as a full time job, liposuction and lipoaugmentation, hand surgery including wrist and distal radius, vascularized composite allograft transplantation, and craniofacial surgery. They would be amused to learn that after all the high tech introductions of lasers, mechanical peels, and alternative chemical peels, nothing works better for skin resurfacing than the old phenol peel with the classic Baker formula. They would smile at the ups and downs of the facelift literature, and feel some pride, I am sure, in learning that it is largely still best as they taught it to us with a SMAS and skin tightening, I was so lucky to fall under the spell of plastic surgery.[1]

Paul Izenberg discussed the changes he witnessed:

> Reflecting back on the late 1970s and early 1980s, it was a time when plastic surgery was changing from a limited array of operative procedures to numerous new approaches to difficult problems allowing innovation—from the fairly standard facelift, rhinoplasty, pressure sore care, random pattern flaps to open rhinoplasty, multiple plane facelifts, musculocutaneous flaps, microvascular surgery, bone plating, subpectoral augmentation, and the beginnings of breast reconstruction. These are just a few of the innovations that began then and progressed to the present amazing field of which we're all now involved.[2]

Ernie Manders added,

> To this day, I am stunned to recall how young the rest our staff was! In retrospect, they were not much older than us. They knew a lot, though, and taught with a pleasure that I remember today. Drs. Bob Oneal, Hack Newman, John Markley, Dennis Bucko, and Paul Izenberg were simply excellent. They were then joined by Eric Austad and Lou Argenta. Each had a special interest to share. I still think of Dennis Bucko and his lessons on oculoplastic surgery. Building on what he taught us, I have done quite a bit of this work with great satisfaction. And I have taught it to keep the flame alive within plastic surgery.[3]

Bruce Novark in 2010 wrote,

> This brings back a lot of memories. We worked hard, learned a lot, and there are many cherished memories.[4]

Bruce sent some additional thoughts in 2015:

> What a great experience it was: surrounded by a wealth of fine faculty and a challenging patient population. We worked hard but never felt mistreated or demeaned; a sense of real collegiality prevailed between the residents and faculty.[5]

Larry Berkowitz commented on his impression of plastic surgery in Ann Arbor:

> I will say that Ann Arbor provided some of the most productive individuals in both the academic and private realm. The number

of lives that were improved and touched by that endeavor must be immeasurable. There will always be those who contribute more than others. Despite tens of thousands of operative procedures, I always wished that I could have left behind a legacy of well-trained, ethically endowed individuals as you (the professors) have done. It is better than a textbook or an instrument with your name on it.[6]

Tom Hudak reflected on the importance of his training:

I will always be grateful for the time that I spent at the University of Michigan. It was very special. We always had plenty of input from the staff and the residents. All of the people in the program at that time were well-trained surgeons and that provided a stimulating atmosphere for learning. On the whole, I thought the program prepared us well for applying our skills in the outside world. I am not sure that everyone enjoyed taping splints or taking out the mail. We were weak in our cleft-lip training and strong in the maxillofacial area. Bob, you were always available for consultation and Lauralee was a good sounding board for the residents' complaints.[7]

Richard Anderson sent his very personal reflection:

You may recall that I had practiced otolaryngology for 10 years and had been thinking about taking a plastic surgery residency for several years. I did interview for a position with Jack Anderson, a then well-known facial plastic and rhinoplasty surgeon in New Orleans. Jack advised me to do a "real" Plastic Surgery residency like Jack Gunter did at Michigan. Later, I did interview for a plastic residency position at Michigan in 1982, as you may recall, and Dick Pollock was chosen that year. After that I was very fortunate to visit with Paul Izenberg and Dr. Dingman at a cosmetic surgery meeting in Birmingham, and they both advised me to put my name in again for a residency position in 1983. I did and the rest is history. Was I lucky or what![8]

Ron Wexler added his impressions:

Every day in my residency was a day of revelation. Everyday brought new problems and answers. Every day I felt that I am improving my skills as a surgeon under the guidance of my teachers . . . this was a stimulating experience.[9]

Issac Peled recalled why he chose Ann Arbor for his fellowship:

> After completing my training as a plastic surgeon and in the military service and against the opinion of the chairman of the department where I trained in Tel Aviv, I decided to apply for a clinical fellowship [even though] my chief considered that I was well trained. Getting to know personally Dingman and Grabb was like being introduced to the "real ones" whom I knew only from reading. I was impressed by the level and the friendliness of the staff including the residents who were carefully chosen and reached key positions in our profession.[10]

## Rounds and Conferences

Lenny Glass recollected,

> Weekly bedside rounds were great, too bad it has, I guess, disappeared in most places [programs]. Trauma [teaching] great for its time, much of it today is obsolete, but then, it was state of the art.[11]

The Thursday teaching conference remains a positive factor for Richard Anderson:

> The Thursday morning [conferences] sessions were always educational, often exciting, and memorable. I was impressed that you [Oneal], John, Paul, Hack, and sometimes Eric were there and contributed so much to the meetings, along with Lou, Tom, Dr. Dingman, Steve Mathes [one year] and other full time dept. staff. Actually, the entire teaching staff was outstanding and amazing.[12]

Paul Izenberg commented on the challenges for the junior residents:

> These conferences were a little nerve wracking for the junior residents as the seniors presented difficult or up and coming patients for an operation and the juniors knew they would have to answer all the questions from the attendings. We all survived it but at times it was an uneasy feeling.[13]

The Saturday bedside rounds left positive memories for Grant Fairbanks:

> One will never forget the Saturday walking rounds at the university hospital large open wards with many beds. One Saturday morning, Dr. Dingman was being asked many questions regarding one patient or another. It was the usual long entourage of residents, interns, and

medical students but on this particular day, Dr. Dingman was in a hurry to be somewhere else. He finally stopped and made a simple but profound directive which covered all options. He turned and said, "Review the situation and do what needs to be done." He then made his exit. In that simple directive, he demonstrated his confidence in his plastic surgery resident team and their ability (already trained general surgeons), to recognize problems for what they were and solve them. Although we valued his knowledge and advice, we didn't need to be "spoon fed." His advice served me and others well for what lay ahead.[14]

## Resident Selection Experiences with Dr. Dingman (ROD)

Jim Stilwell (Saint Joseph Mercy Hospital [SJMH] plastic surgery resident, 1960–62) recalled the "procedure" for selecting residents circa 1960:

> My favorite memory is how I got to be a resident in Dr. Dingman's program. In the spring of 1960, I was a third-year resident in surgery at the Medical University of South Carolina in Charleston and was working with Dr. Robert Hagerty in the lab. Dr. Hagerty called me one day to get down to the auditorium to hear Dr. Dingman as visiting professor speak to a large group of doctors. I spent the next thirty minutes listening to the most fascinating program with slides that I had ever heard. Afterwards, I told Dr. Hagerty I wanted to be in Dr. Dingman's program and he said, "I thought you would." He then invited me to his home to meet Dr. Dingman. During the evening, Dr. Dingman made an appointment for me to meet him at the Ann Arbor VA Hospital two days later. I flew up to Ann Arbor the next day, met and scrubbed with him and answered his questions for about eight hours. He then took me to his home, made me a Scotch and soda, and introduced me to his wife and Bill Grabb. On the way back to my hotel, he stopped the car and looked at me for a very long time and then said, "Jim—I guess you have got the job. But you have got to learn to speak English!!" I flew back to Charleston, worked on my drawl, and started at SJMH in July, 1960.[15]

A recollection from Dr. Jim Norris offers additional insight into Dr. Dingman's character and judgment about selecting residents. In 1971, Jim, who was black, had applied to two other residency programs in addition to the University of Michigan (UM). He sent his application to one and they asked for a photograph, which he sent, and he never heard from them again. He applied to another one of the New York hospitals, and he was not even offered an interview. Jim continued,

Contrast that with the hospitality shown on my interview with Dr. Dingman in Ann Arbor. I was invited to go on rounds with him and in his office afterwards he sat down one on one with me and said, "I would like very much to have you join our program." He was aware that I was going to Northwestern for an interview with Dr. B. Herold Griffith and he suggested I take a week or two to think things over. A week later he called me at Tuskegee to find out how things had gone at Northwestern. I told him it went well. He said, "I know you were concerned about experience in head and neck surgery, but I believe we can offer you adequate training in that. I just wanted to reassure you."[16]

It is to be noted that the help Dr. Dingman was willing to provide when residents finished the training program was just as significant. Jim, who wanted to relocate to New York City (NYC), recalled Dr. Dingman's willingness to speak to some of his colleagues on Jim's behalf before Jim's visit there. Jim recollected that during the visit several interviews resulted only in an offer for a rather minor position at Harlem Hospital with no other hospital affiliation. When Jim came back to Ann Arbor, Dr. Dingman wanted to know all about his visit to NYC. Jim described this meeting:

When I returned to Michigan I saw Dr. Dingman at Mott Hospital. He was preparing to operate on a child and he turned to me and said, "Jim, how did things go with you in New York City?" I related my experiences, particularly with the most egregious circumstance. Dr. Dingman turned beet red in the face, poked a finger in my chest and said, "Look, if you want to go up to New York City and work at Harlem Hospital that is your decision, but don't let those New York fellows put you in a box and label you as a black plastic surgeon. You are as well trained as any plastic surgeon in New York."[17]

This quote really says a lot about Dr. Dingman and his acceptance and promoting of his trainees based on their character and performance.

## Dr. Dingman's Outside Activities beyond His Plastic Surgery Practice

Dr. Dingman loved hunting of all varieties. He made many trips with friends including big game hunting. He loved duck hunting in Canada and fishing in Lake Michigan. Ernie Manders recalled,

Dr. Dingman had incredible stamina. On one day in the OR doing an all-day aesthetic case, we neared the end at about three in the

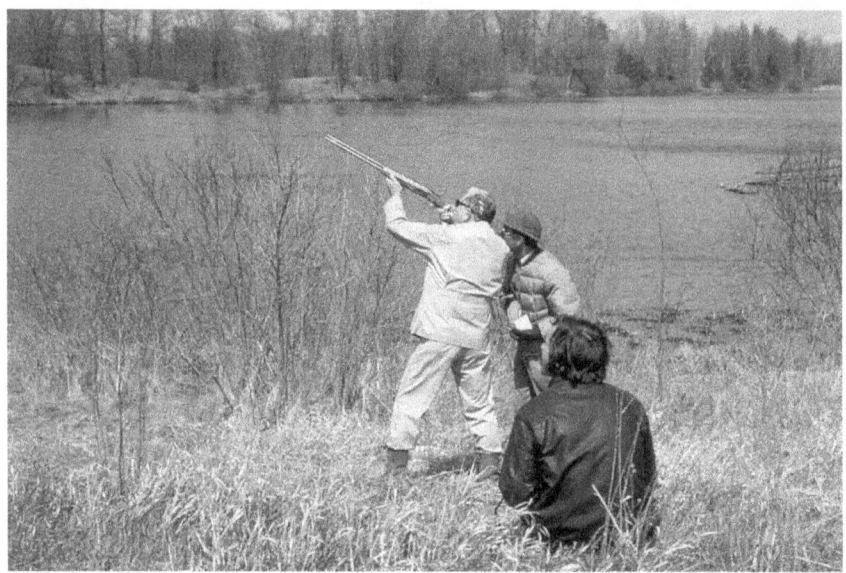

*Photo 64:* Dr. Dingman duck hunting.

afternoon. Dr. Dingman said, "Ernie, I have to go duck hunting on the Indian reservation in Canada. Can you finish up?" "Yes, Sir, I said." The next day on coming down to the OR here was Dr. Dingman as usual sitting in a dictation cubbyhole and reviewing his charts for the patients that day. "Ernie" he chimed, "great hunting yesterday. Bunch of ducks for you in the freezer in the nursing station on Fourth Floor" [Photo 64].[18]

Lauralee remembered,

In the spring Dr. Dingman brought me peonies from his garden. He would fill our bathroom sink in the office with water and put the flowers in and then he would leave me a note "look in the bathroom sink."

She also recollected another adventure. Dr. Dingman loved taking photographs and always had a camera ready for all occasions:

One morning I put on a tape from ROD and was very surprised. He announced he was dictating from the roof of his home on Chestnut Road so he could record leaks and flaws in his rubber roof. Just the idea that he was walking around on his roof scared me. My function was to faithfully transcribe this inspection so that he could talk to the roofing company, lawyer, or whoever came to check it out [Photo 65].[19]

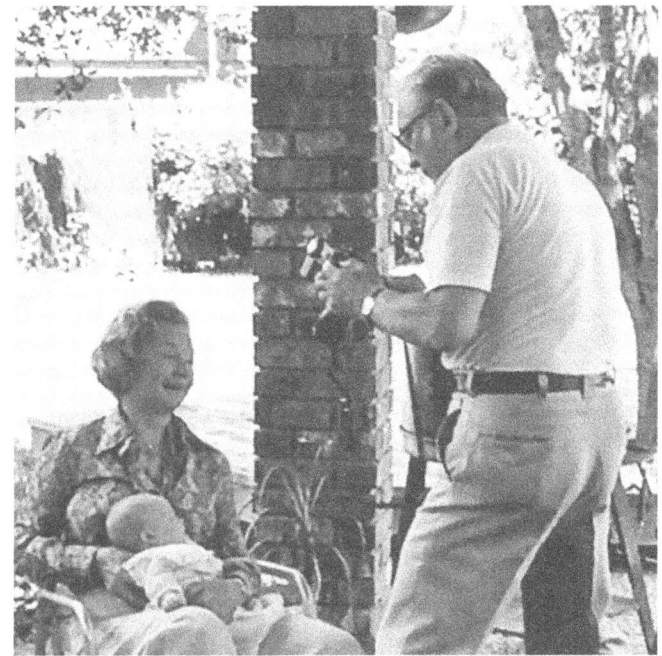

*Photo 65:* Dr. Dingman photographing Mrs. Dingman holding Dr. Cromwell's baby, with his ever-ready camera.

## ROD's Personal Anecdotes/Adages

Bob Wilensky recollected Dr. Dingman's adages such as "if you take a pig with loose skin and tighten the skin you have a pig with tight skin" and "you can't turn a peach into a carrot."[20] Ted Dodenhoff recalled ROD's farewell advice as Ted set off to begin a practice: "He walked me out to the car, shook my hand, and with his usual modest demeanor said, 'Ted, I'm sure you will be successful. You've had the finest training in Plastic Surgery that exists anywhere in the world.' The perfect finish."[21] Several of the residents who had come from other countries admired his style. Ron Wexler wrote,

> Napoleon said, "every soldier carries in his backpack the Baton de Marechal" (a symbol of dignity) . . . this famous saying came to my mind once when I came to ROD's office and saw him sitting with his two legs on the table and on the opposite side of the table, one of our medical students with his legs on the same table too . . . and these two people, the world famous professor on one side and the medical rookie on the other were discussing . . . something. This is a view you could see then only in America.[22]

## Importance of Photography to Dr. Dingman

Jim Norris related,

> Every annual meeting of the ASPS Dr. Dingman would prepare his exhibit on "Plastic Surgeons I have known." I believe I helped him set up the exhibit almost every year from 1973 until Dr. Dingman no longer attended the meetings. Afterwards, we would set up the carousel and then put it on timed exposure, we would sit down and run through the carousel about twice. I thought this was a really neat part of his photography hobby, but now I think that Dr. Dingman had another motive for putting on that exhibit. In that way, he could refresh his memory about all the faces of plastic surgeons he had known. Maybe I am wrong, but I recall his colleagues were often amazed that he had total recall of their names.[23]

Lauralee recalled,

> Dr. Dingman loved to take pictures and then to review the slides on his light board table he had in the basement of his office. He had thousands of before and after patient slides suitable for teaching residents but also for lecturing at meetings. His dictum was "you can never take too many slides." Dr. Dingman felt that a certain shade of blue wool fabric was an ideal background for his photographs and only one store in Ann Arbor (Fabers Department Store) had this exact shade of blue. Every resident and staff had a large piece of this fabric folded in his camera case, as important as a roll of film [Photo 66].[24]

Dr. Louis Mes observed, shortly after he began his residency, that Dr. Dingman was quite a stickler about his photographs:

> Shortly after I joined the residency program and began with the SJMH rotation, he called me into his office one day and quietly asked me if I had taken the pictures that he had spread over his desk in front of him. Proudly, I assured him that I had and waited for his praise. Instead, without saying a word he picked up the trash can next to the desk and swept the lot into it. He did not look up and I slid out of there with my ego in tatters. The matter was never raised again and my photography skills improved exponentially within 24 hours. That is why we respected him and worked so hard for him.[25]

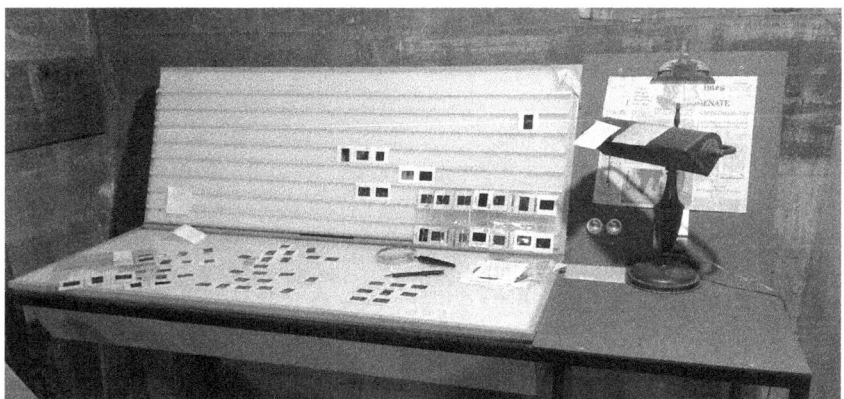

Photo 66: Dr. Dingman's light board table for reviewing and labeling slides, which was later gifted to Dr. Oneal and now in his basement study.

Bob Wilensky, early on, learned another important requirement for photography:

> Dr. Dingman insisted that a photograph should never be taken that was not suitable for presentation at a national meeting. Clean towels around the wound, no blood in the field, patients face not showing if it was not part of the operative field. He also insisted on patients not having makeup if that was possible or at least having the photographs match pre and post operatively with hairstyles, makeup and so forth.[26]

## Graduations

Grant Fairbanks recalled the significance of an informal graduation ceremony:

> Graduation from the Plastic Surgery program in 1971 was without great fanfare. Dr. Dingman invited Carl Berner and myself to a small restaurant on the west side of downtown Ann Arbor [most likely the Town Club] where the three of us had lunch together. He presented us with a certificate signed by himself and Director of University Hospital as well as Chairman of the Surgery Department. There were no speeches and no fanfare, but the strength and warmth of Dr. Dingman's personality was pervasive. He gave us both a signed photograph of himself—his classic one—inscripted with "Best Wishes Reed O. Dingman, M.D." We were now full-fledged Plastic Surgeons approved by our Chief. It was enough of a sendoff.[27]

## Another Memorable Event

One of the most frightening operating room events for Lenny Glass turned out to be a result of his wartime Vietnam experience. Just prior to beginning the residency in Ann Arbor, Lenny was in the army as a surgeon and stationed in Vietnam for a year. While there in an outpost, his unit was shelled by the Viet Cong many times at night, and he learned to seek cover reflexively, usually under his cot. In his first year of residency, he and I were operating together on a cleft lip patient at SJMH. In those days, the surgical field suction apparatus was connected to a large glass bottle under the head of the table. Suddenly, the bottle imploded, and it sounded just like a bomb. I looked up, and Lenny, across the table from me, had completely vanished. In a few moments, he reappeared having reflexly dived under the operating table.[28]

## Memories of Visiting Professors

The UM residency training program benefited from a large number of very distinguished visiting professors. As Grant Fairbanks wrote,

> Dr. Dingman was able to attract excellent visiting professors for our program. One such person was Mr. John C. Mustarde from Scotland, an MD trained in both plastic surgery and ophthalmology, who had written an authoritative textbook on ophthalmic plastic surgery. Dr. Dingman asked me to serve as a part-time chauffeur for Mr. Mustarde, and Carl Berner, my residency mate, was the other chauffeur. One of us picked him up at Detroit Metro Airport and the other delivered him back. Such personal contact with Mr. Mustarde was a highlight. He signed my copy of his book with reference to me as his chauffeur. He gave us some profound insights into ophthalmic plastic surgery, which would serve us well.[29]

Issac Peled recollected John Mustarde from another trip as visiting professor: "Dingman invited John Mustarde and he was operating at SJMH while I was his assistant in an eyelid reconstruction. One of the kibitzers kicked my ankle and when I looked at him, he whispered in my ear 'call him Mr. not Dr,' and this was also a lesson."[30]

Don Greer shared his experience of having the visiting professor present on a Saturday: "The most impressive memory of those rounds is of the visiting professor offering a new and insightful and usually helpful comments on every single patient. It was an awesome display of clinical knowledge from a surgeon far out of his usual field of practice."[31]

## About Dr. William C. Grabb (WCG)

Bruce Novark remembered Bill Grabb as the "consummate organizer, thinker, administrator, and author—a whirlwind of academic activity"[32] Grabb's leadership is recalled by Ernie Manders: "Dr. Grabb was very much involved in the leadership of organized and academic plastic surgery." He also remembered his own first face-lift procedure as a senior resident undertaken with Grabb's supervision.

> I took my place on the right side of the table. Dr. Grabb was concentrating on doing paperwork, reading galleys, editing them, and even dictating notes in the corner. "Go ahead," he said. I must confess that I did somewhat resent the fact that the master was not carefully watching my every move. Later I understood the message: "You can do it and we trained YOU to do it!" It has informed my teaching [philosophy] on our reconstructive service at Pittsburgh. Another important lesson he taught was to champion others with good ideas. It was he who stood up and wrote a supporting commentary for Dr. Chedomir Radovan's first paper on tissue expansion. He helped get him on national programs. He invited him to Michigan. Due in part to Dr. Eric Austad's brilliant innovation of tissue expansion with an osmotic expander, Dr. Grabb's mind was open to the idea of tissue expansion long before any of his contemporaries.[33]

Lauralee recollected that Dr. Grabb enjoyed writing and editing books and articles concerned with plastic surgery education. He published several texts, was an excellent editor, and wrote many journal articles but always found time for outside activities. He was a devoted sailor and raced a Snipe almost every Sunday afternoon at Barton Pond; in winter, he occasionally sailed an ice boat, close to the icy edge. He also crewed for friends on much larger boats in the Detroit to Mackinaw race almost every year. Besides these activities, he was a hot-air balloonist, the first one with a license in Michigan. He received his inspiration at a party at the Oneal's home where he admired Zibby's collection of paintings of eighteenth-century hot-air balloon ascensions. "On one weekend, he went to South Dakota to learn how. His balloon was red, white, and blue and named 'the Yankee Doodle' (see Photo 67). It was a one-man balloon and had no basket. It had just a seat like a swing"[34] (see Photo 68). Someone, usually one of his family members, would have to track him, whichever way the wind was blowing and follow him until he landed, occasionally in a corn field, to pick him and the balloon up. Lauralee recalled, "He sponsored many balloon ascensions from a field near his home and frequently entertained all the members

138  *Reflections and Commentary*

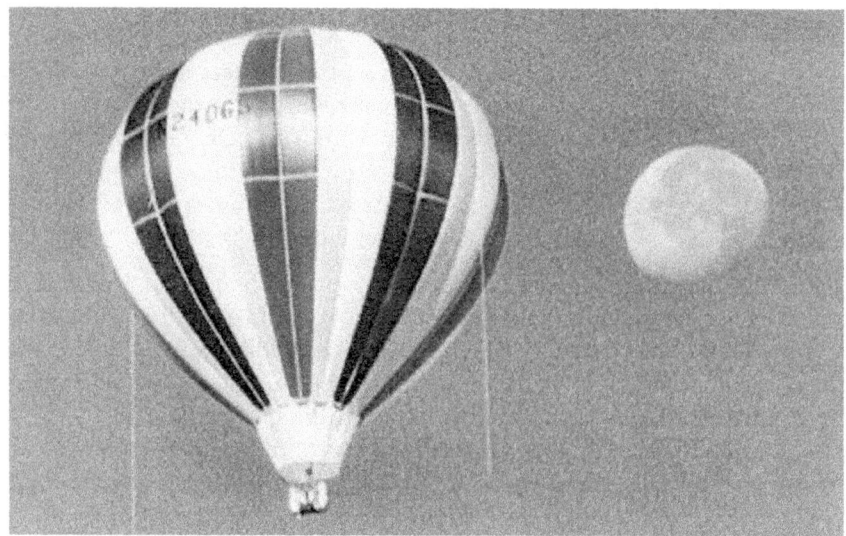

*Photo 67:* Yankee Doodle, Bill Grabb's balloon.

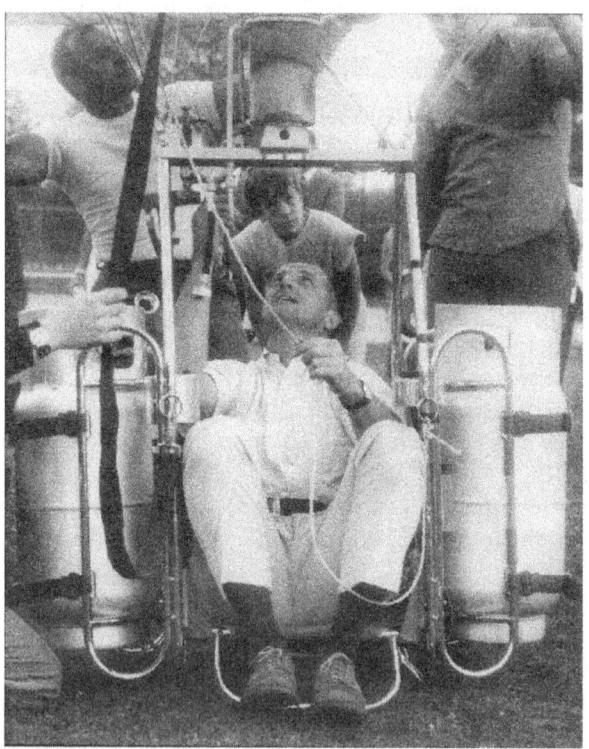

*Photo 68:* Bill in the seat of the balloon.

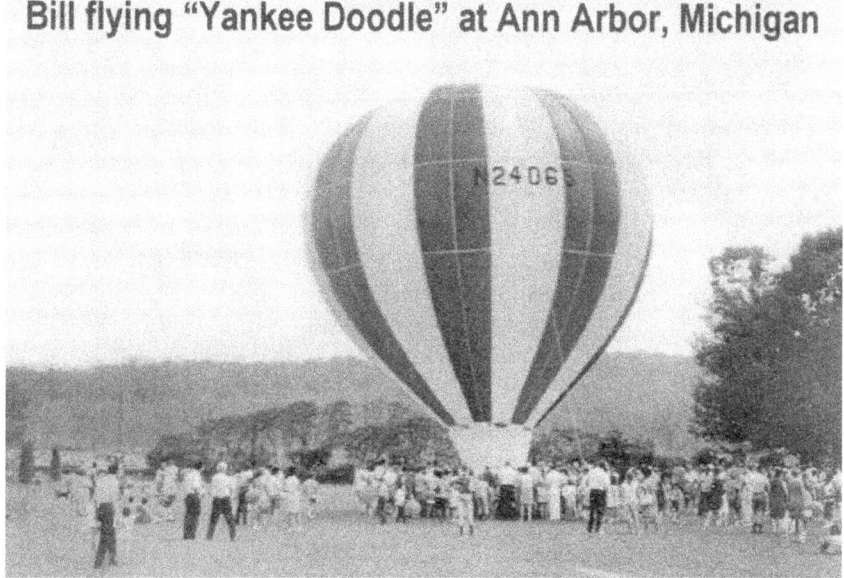

Photo 69: Balloon launching party from a field near Grabb's house in Ann Arbor.

of the Section of Plastic Surgery and their friends and wives for very festive afternoons"[35] (see Photo 69). Ballooning became quite a passion for Bill who had a love of flying even before his tenure in the US Air Force. When Dr. Millard asked him whether he wrote his books while in the air, he admitted, "No, once up, I spend most of my time figuring how to get back down!"[36] He began to spend summer vacations with his family at the US National Hot Air Balloon Championships, and in 1971–73, he served as president of the Balloon Federation of America during which, in 1972, he flew over the Alps in Switzerland in a two-man balloon. In 1978, he flew over the US continental divide in a gas balloon with two other pilots, and in 1980, he participated in the XIII Winter Olympics in Lake Placid, New York, by flying over the stadium. He was inducted posthumously into the US Ballooning Hall of Fame in 2012.

The comments that follow were selected from Malcolm Marks's Grabb Lecture at the ROD Society meeting in 2007 in Ann Arbor.

He first spoke about his admiration for Bill Grabb as well as Bill's many talents: "Bill Grabb created for us a unique atmosphere for academic pursuits that was stimulating, challenging, and pleasurable. His great talent for teaching set an example in humility and honesty, which will always remain dear to us. We are extremely honored to have had the privilege of studying with such a kind and knowledgeable man."[37]

He then spoke honoring the recent retirements of Drs. Newman, Markley, and Oneal:

> I have deep respect and admiration for those I talk about today as well as the respect and admiration for this program. Those I talk about have helped shape the way I think, teach, and live and I am forever grateful.
>
> There is a group of us who have been educated by all of those we honor today: doctors Dingman, Grabb, Oneal, Markley, and Newman and that group is the bridge from the past to the present for several teaching programs in the United States. With the retirement of Drs. Oneal, Markley, and Newman, an era is coming to an end. These are the guys who helped build the foundation of what is undoubtedly one of the most prominent programs in America. They are the people who helped guide this program through difficult and tumultuous stages. They are the people who were here when others were leaving and others were coming and every resident who has trained here for over thirty years owes them a debt of gratitude.
>
> Hack Newman, with all his knowledge and talent, always made you understand that he felt privileged to be able to teach. He brought to the plastic surgery department the knowledge and approach of a veteran otolaryngologist. He has been recognized nationally and internationally for his expertise in rhinoplasty and has been an invited speaker for a multitude of courses and panels. He was honored by his fellow plastic surgeons in Michigan serving as their society's president for two years. Dr. Newman has the unique ability to make everyone feel like his friend. I fondly remember being invited to their home shortly before graduation along with Bob Gilman and Glen Harder for dinner and samples of wine that I either didn't know about or couldn't afford at the time. I never saw him angry, upset, or frustrated no matter what we did or didn't do. He shared his skill in pediatric, craniofacial, cosmetic, and head and neck surgery and taught a lot more than just medicine. His joy and love of life is contagious.
>
> John Markley has proven that in the right environment, an environment that as I said makes this program so special, you could have a successful private practice and as well as pursue a career-long involvement in teaching and research. We all know that John initiated the research with Dr. Faulkner that is going on today, was the lone microsurgeon in the early days of microsurgery here, and continued to develop technical and intellectual skills that few of us can achieve.

He was writing articles related to skeletal muscle adaptation and facial nerve paralysis thirty years ago and was one of the first to write about neurovascular tissue transfer. What amazed me about Dr. Markley when I was a young resident was how someone could be so smart and still be in such good shape. I was used to meeting the occasional person who was one or the other, but not both. He is as knowledgeable a hand surgeon as one can be and has shared his knowledge with countless young surgeons over a very long career. He taught the importance of anatomy and attention to detail while moving forward efficiently. He did this at the same time he ran his practice and maintained a level of physical condition that enables him to pursue and enjoy athletic skills at an age that most people are beginning to take things easy. Despite what he might say, I have no doubt that his kayaking is already at a high level.

Bob Oneal is a man who has had as great an impact on me as any man I have had the privilege to work with. He too has spent a huge part of his professional life teaching because of his love of our profession and his love for teaching. I still remember the hours that he and Paul Izenberg spent dissecting cadavers, learning every possible detail about the anatomy of the face and later the nose in preparation for the Dallas Rhinoplasty course. Over the course of his career, he has at different times become an expert in cleft lip and palate, breast surgery, facial aesthetic surgery, anatomy of the face, and rhinoplasty. As a resident, it was Dr. Oneal as much as anyone who made me want to learn more about something than I really needed to know. His general knowledge about everything related to plastic surgery made me want to read more. He taught me not to be satisfied with less than the absolute best you can achieve and to be savagely critical of your work and results. He taught me the importance of humility, and along with Drs. Grabb and Argenta, it was his influence that made me want to stay in the university environment.[38]

Lauralee observed (and she insisted the following remarks about me be included),

> Bob Oneal is humble by nature and a worrier by experience. While we were working on this book, he often worried about praise directed to himself. He felt that favorable remarks for him shouldn't be included as it was immodest. I told him the combo was always Dingman/Grabb/Oneal and he couldn't be left out. Residents often mentioned that Bob was a favorite (or THE favorite) and I think I know why. Bob never forgot how he felt during his residency. It was natural

for him to be sympathetic and fraternal, especially during times of overwork and stress. I believe he chose the necessary but difficult role as Resident Advocate and friend as his major contribution to the success of the program—and no one did it better.[39]

Bruce Novark called Oneal his favorite teacher: "He always inspired me to analyze and think about the surgical problem at hand, to consider the various possibilities and approaches to solution. He would discuss the advantages and disadvantages—his experience and that of others with each prospective procedure. Others would say or imply: 'this is how I do it.' Certainly I learned from those experiences, but not as much or as productively as when Bob was the teacher. He then always demonstrated great and kind patience in guiding the neophyte surgeon through the exercise. His influence 'stuck.'"[40] Issac Peled wrote, "Working and socializing with Bob was a great pleasure, although he thought that I couldn't stand his surgical rhythm, it took longer than others but I heard and learned from him besides the meticulous performance that 'in six months' time nobody will ask how long did the surgery take.'"[41]

Grant Fairbanks added, "Bob Oneal was always there for the residents. Bob's constancy and his unwavering loyalty to the program, to ROD and WCG and to the residents in training, left an indelible impression on me."[42]

## About Lauralee Lutz

In her own words, Lauralee described more memories and experiences:

> ROD thought I was in charge of everything. He would announce "there are no hand towels in the men's room" and I had to figure out how to get them or "can you arrange to have these windows washed." My answer was always "**Yes**" and I would figure out later how to do it. One of ROD's favorite lunches in the hospital cafeteria was a hardboiled egg and a dish of cottage cheese. When residents joined the service, he reminded them not to discuss patients while in the food line or in the elevators as you never know when the relatives were going to be there. Good advice. Dr. Dingman always had a great day when Mr. Kilgore from Coldwater, Michigan, would show up. He sold human skulls (we think he dug them up in Mexico). Lou Argenta and ROD always chose the most abnormal skulls for their personal collection. For several years, ROD gave each graduating resident a real human skull in a black box. The residents considered this the best possible gift. I think this might be illegal now, so plastic skulls are on the market.[43]

Bruce Novark observed, "Lauralee was our angel in the office next door, our literary leprechaun. She was always the faculty's right hand and resident's knowledgeable buddy, helper, and encyclopedia on U of M Plastic Surgery—and Shakespeare."[44] According to Issac Peled, "It didn't take me much time to realize that the Section was directed by Bill but organized by L3. She had the answers to almost everything and would take care of any single detail. I am pretty sure that all of us would have taken L3 as 'charge d'affaires' of our practice and managing our department."[45] In 1984, Lauralee published "Shakespeare on Plastic Surgery" in the *Plastic and Reconstructive Surgery* journal, where she recorded fifteen quotes related to various aspects and procedures in plastic surgery: "Allow not more than nature needs" (*King Lear*, act 2, sc. 4) as applied to reduction mammoplasty is an example of her familiarity with the Bard but also her understanding the many aspects of our specialty.[46] Ernie Manders recollected Lauralee quoting the Bard, "How poor is he who hath not patience. What wound didst ever heal but by degrees?" and then ends by saying: "I have searched for 35 years for another Lauralee and I have learned THERE IS ONLY ONE!"[47]

## To Conclude . . . a Potpurii of Memories and Reflections of Dr. Dingman

From the early 1960s to 1976, the first-year resident at Ford rotated for six months at SJMH in Ann Arbor to gain more pediatric and cosmetic surgery experience. These residents shared call and day-to-day patient responsibilities with the UM resident rotating through St. Joe and were considered integral participants in the training program. Don Ditmars (Henry Ford Hospital [HFH] rotator, 1970) reflected on his impressions and recollection of his training experience in Ann Arbor:

> In the middle of the 1960s, Henry Ford Hospital plastic surgery residents began rotating with Dr. Dingman at St. Joseph Mercy Hospital in Ann Arbor for six months. During this time, they were responsible for every patient in the operating room and also were in Dr. Dingman's office for pre- and postoperative evaluations and care. These were primarily cosmetic patients. However, the Henry Ford residents also were involved with Dr. William Grabb's patients, which were mostly reconstructive cases. Dr. Robert Oneal joined this group at the latter part of the decade. As one of those residents, I realize that I got more from that rotation than just observing the masters at work. We learned how to interact with cosmetic patients. The concept of backing up our work with free revisions as necessary was part and parcel of this very effective interaction. We were involved

with the preoperative planning, which was sometimes innovative and always involved medical photography. The use and composition of standard photography for rhinoplasty was invaluable. Almost of equal importance, this was our first interaction with medical students who were eager to learn. Becoming effective teachers was part of our experience at the time, which stayed with us when we returned home to Henry Ford Hospital to complete our residency and then as we went into practice. In summary, it was a real privilege to be able to be with a true early Master in Plastic Surgery.[48]

Don Greer observed, "On the very last day of my residency, as a going away present, I was given permission to assist Dr. Dingman on one of his cases, which happened to be a rhinoplasty, on a lady physician. Halfway through the case, things started going badly. The room became very quiet. And then even quieter. Time really dragged. Several options were tried, and finally an acceptable result appeared. We were all glad to flee the room. On the way out, Dr. Dingman draped an arm on my shoulder, and commented 'Always remember that problems can occur to anyone!'"[49]

Bruce Novark recollected "that Lauralee called Dr. Dingman 'our gentle giant.' I remember him as a true gentleman, a giant in the world of plastic surgery and like a father. My father (a tool and die maker) was killed in an auto accident when I was 4 years old. Boys growing up without a dad spend years searching for a 'father' a role model, a great mentor. I finally found mine in Dr. Dingman."[50] Several of the residents saw Dr. Dingman this way. Jim Norris wrote, "Dr. Dingman is the one man that I felt was more like my father than any man I worked with."[51] Grant Fairbanks agreed, "Without question, Dr. Dingman was a second father to all his residents. He was admired and revered by all." Fairbanks went on to say, "To receive the private verbal approval of our professor, Reed O Dingman, meant more than any medal, certificate, public honor, or applause. It just made one to want to work harder and strive for greater perfection. In the operating room, Dr. Dingman demonstrated consummate skill. He would give his residents responsibility to the extent he felt they were capable, and frequently more, to allow for their growth. We never wanted to disappoint him. He seemed to inherently know each resident's limits."[52]

The following are selected passages from recollections of Harvey Weiss (HFH rotator, 1966):

During my first year of plastic surgery residency, I rotated through Dr. Dingman's private service at St. Joseph Mercy Hospital in Ann Arbor. We operated with him almost every weekday. The operating room was always filled with visiting professors and other interested plastic surgeons who wanted to see the latest techniques.

Dr. Dingman never, to my knowledge, refused any qualified surgeon an audience. The conversations were continuous, spirited, philosophical, practical, and ranged from medicine to sports. He always included the students and nurses. In the operating room, he rarely backtracked and even though he seemed to be moving slowly, there were no wasted motions—a valuable lesson in the O.R. and in life! I wish recent and current residents could have had the privilege of working with this truly remarkable mentor.[53]

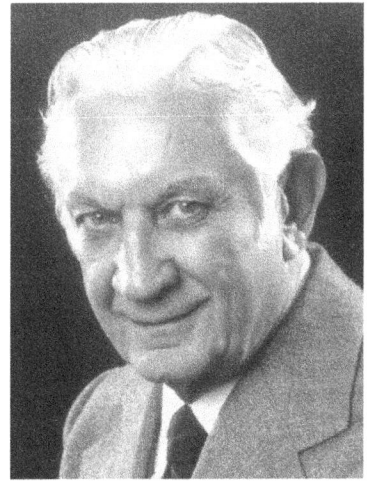

Photo 70: Dr. Reed O. Dingman.

As demonstrated by these comments, we all, myself and Lauralee and all the contributors, feel fortunate to have had such a fruitful and meaningful relationship as student, resident, associate, and friend with someone of Dr. Dingman's energy, vision, and genius. Like so many others who trained and worked with Dr. Dingman, we felt that he was bigger than life and absolutely the most important influence in our professional lives (Photo 70).

# Epilogue

While Dr. Argenta was the acting head of the Section of Plastic Surgery from 1985 to 1986, a search committee was again appointed to recommend to the chairman of the Department of Surgery a candidate for the permanent head of the Section of Plastic Surgery. The committee had wide representation from within the Department of Surgery including myself. After interviewing several candidates for this position, there was strong support for Lou Argenta. The committee admired Lou for his leadership abilities, his commitment to education, and his wide-ranging research accomplishments, in addition to his well-known surgical skills. Lou had the support of the faculty and staff of the plastic surgery section as well. He was recognized for his long-standing loyalty to the University of Michigan (UM) Medical School. By the time the actual selection was made, Dr. Turcotte had retired as head of the Department of Surgery and Dr. Laser Greenfield had assumed that position. He chose Dr. David Smith to be the new section head of plastic surgery starting July of 1987.

Soon after his appointment, at my invitation, Dr. Smith and I met at my house in Ann Arbor. The purpose of the visit was to welcome him and to be sure he was fully aware of the details of the long-standing affiliation between faculty at Saint Joseph Mercy Hospital (SJMH) and the UM resident training program and the fact that the residency actually originated there. After the section was formed at UM, the residents continued to rotate to SJMH. I wanted to emphasize the importance we had all felt about the quality of the preceptorship experience at SJMH as well as the positive responses we had from the vast majority of the residents about their rotations at SJMH. I think this discussion was invaluable for the maintaining of the affiliation, and SJMH still remains in the residents' rotation schedule. Of additional significance for the UM program is that the affiliation with the plastic surgery program at SJMH has continued in an uninterrupted and integrated fashion for all these fifty-two years since the UM section was formed. It now serves as a rotation for two residents for two months twice during their training, thus mutually enhancing the lives of both the adjunct faculty at SJMH and the residents in training.

In 1983, Dr. Malcolm Marks had left the UM faculty for three years to be on the Tulane faculty but returned to UM again to join Dr. Argenta on the faculty between 1986 and 1988 and to participate in research activities at that time. Malcolm related to me about that time period on the faculty here at Michigan: "That period on faculty working with Drs. Argenta and Stevenson and for a short time with Dr. Smith was an exciting and educational experience. We were very busy in all areas of plastic surgery. We were integral in establishing the multidisciplinary breast [clinic] during that time. I was fortunate to experience a period of transition from the Dingman/Grabb era to the present program."[1] In 1988, Dr. Marks left with Dr. Argenta to Bowman Gray Medical Center where Dr. Argenta assumed the chairmanship of plastic surgery and Malcolm is now chairman. His recent personal reflection follows: "I believe the education and experiences at the University of Michigan have contributed immensely to the success of the Plastic Surgery department at Wake Forest as it has to the multitude of programs and practices of alumni around the country. I am forever grateful to the faculty and residents with whom I was associated in those years as well as to Lauralee and the staff who were so important in my daily life at that time."[2]

The two cleft palate clinics, at SJMH and the UM, functioned somewhat independently even after Dr. Smith became the section head. After much discussion by all parties concerned in the mid-1980s and by mutual agreement, the SJMH clinic was terminated and all of our private cleft lip and palate patients were seen regularly in the clinic at UM. There was the additional advantage in that the SJMH faculty were able to perform our surgical procedures on their private patients, especially on infants, at UM where pediatric anesthesiologists and a pediatric intensive care unit were available.

Under Dr. Smith's leadership, the program grew with the addition of more permanent faculty and expansion of the hand and craniofacial programs, and eventually, fellowships were offered. Resident training gradually evolved in a totally integrated six-year program accepting potential trainees directly out of medical school, most of whom would spend a year or more either in research or in a variety of master's degree programs. There were still places for the occasional fully boarded general or ENT surgeon.

In 2001, the program continued to thrive under Dr. William Kuzon's leadership as section head. He had joined the UM faculty under Dr. Smith after obtaining a PhD during his plastic surgery training at the University of Toronto. Under his leadership, there were significant increases in both clinical and laboratory research. After Dr. Kuzon's eleven-year tenure, Dr. Paul Cederna, in 2012, became the section head, and under his leadership, further expansion of the faculty in craniofacial, hand, and microvascular surgery occurred as well as continued expansion of the research program. An interesting link with the past is the current ongoing research directed by Dr. Cederna on developing a biologic interface between an amputee's nerve endings and the prosthesis itself. Some of the muscle transfer procedures reflect earlier work from the lab of Dr. John Faulkner and Dr. Bruce Carlson.[3] This work was based partially on the muscle transfer work begun in conjunction with Dr. John Markley in the Faulkner lab (chapter six).

There are currently fifteen active faculty in the section. A very active research program continues. The number of residents was recently expanded from three to four trainees per year. There are currently eighteen residents in clinical rotations and four on lab rotations. Teaching remains an important aspect of the training program. A recent example was the 2014 publication in the second edition of the *Michigan Manual of Plastic Surgery*, a guide to patient care, primarily compiled by our Michigan residents in training with the guidance of the faculty.[4] The program is currently considered one of the top plastic surgery training and research centers in the country.

# Appendix

## A-1. Visiting Plastic Surgery Professors during the Early Years of the University of Michigan Section of Plastic Surgery

**1966–67:** Mr. John Batstone, Oxford, England; Dr. Richard Stark, New York City; Dr. Ralph Millard, Miami; Dr. Ralph Blocksma, Grand Rapids; Drs. James Sullivan and George Baibak, Toledo; Dr. Richard Straith, Detroit; Dr. Robert Pool, Beaumont Hospital, Royal Oak, MI.

**1967–68:** Dr. Paul Pickering, San Diego; Dr. Ken Dorner, Kalamazoo; Dr. J. William Littler, New York City.

**1968–69:** Dr. Herbert Mehnert, Innsbruck, Austria; Dr. Hunter Fry, Melbourne, Australia; Dr. Herold Griffith, Northwestern University, Chicago; Dr. Tom Kendall, University of Kansas, Lawrence; Dr. C. G. Knowles, Lancaster, England.

**1969–70:** Mr. John Mustarde, Glasgow, Scotland. Famous oculoplastic surgeon and author of *Plastic Surgery of the Orbital Region*. He was visiting professor for three days, and he lectured, operated, and reviewed patients.

**1970–71:** Dr. M. Sasaki, Tokyo, Japan (drew the picture of L3); Dr. H. Schule, Stuttgart, Germany; Dr. Wolfgang Muhlbauer, Munich, Germany; Dr. Guellerma Raspall, Barcelona, Spain; Dr. Takehiko Ohura, Hokkaido, Japan

**1971–72:** These visitors were in addition to those participating in the faculty for Plastic Surgery in General Surgery Practice conference. Dr. Stuart Milton, Oxford, England; Dr. Bernard O'Brien, Melbourne, Australia; Dr. Ortiz Monasterio, Mexico City, Mexico.

**1972–73:** Dr. Guerro-Santos, Guadalajara, Mexico.

**1973–74:** The only visitors for that year were the faculty for the postgraduate course "Plastic Surgery in General Surgery Practice": Dr. Paul Weeks, St. Louis; Dr. John Gaisford, Pittsburgh; Dr. Shattuck Hartwell, Cleveland; Dr. George Crickelair, New York City.

## A-2. Plastic Surgery Residency Training in Ann Arbor/Saint Joseph Mercy Hospital (SJMH) and University of Michigan, 1958–86

### Residents and Their Year of Graduation from the Program

SJMH Program

| | |
|---|---|
| Natvig, Paul, MD | 1958 |
| Grabb, William, MD | 1961 |
| Bell, Gordon, MD | 1962 |
| Mauzy, Merritt, MD | 1962 |
| Stilwell, James, MD | 1962 |
| Alger, John, MD | 1963 |
| Au, Otto, MD | 1963 |
| Lucid, Morgan, MD | 1964 |

University of Michigan Section of Plastic Surgery Program
Reed O. Dingman, DDS, MD, Section Head

| | |
|---|---|
| Tipton, John, MD | 1965 |
| Davis, Don G., MD | 1966 |
| Oneal, Robert M., MD | 1966 |
| Knode, Robert, MD | 1967 |
| Russell, Jim, MD | 1967 |
| Chapple, John G., MD | 1968 |
| Constant, Errikos, MD | 1968 |
| Wilms, Fred, MD | 1968 |
| Borocz, Steve, MD | 1969 |
| Dodenhoff, Theodore, MD | 1969 |
| Ramos, Hernando, MD | 1969 |
| Seaton, Ralph, Jr., MD | 1969 |
| Glass, Leonard W., MD | 1970 |
| Hudak, Thomas, MD | 1970 |
| Kloster, Gilbert, MD | 1970 |
| Berner, Carl, MD | 1971 |
| Fairbanks, Grant, MD | 1971 |
| Geisterfer, Dirk, MD | 1972 |
| Greer, Donald, Jr., MD | 1972 |
| Wexler, Menachem, MD | 1972 |
| Cromwell, Terry A., MD | 1973 |

| | |
|---|---|
| Nobel, Gary, MD | 1973 |
| Thorvaldssen, Sigurdur, MD | 1973 |
| Norris, James, MD | 1974 |
| Novark, Bruce, MD, DDS | 1974 |
| O'Connor, John, MD, DDS | 1974 |
| Lawrence, Richard, MD | 1975 |
| MacCollum, Maxwell, MD | 1975 |
| Wilensky, Robert J., MD, PhD | 1975 |
| Agris, Joseph, MD, DDS | 1976 |
| Blackburn, Bill, MD | 1976 |
| Bucko, Dennis, MD | 1976 |

**William C. Grabb, MD, Section Head**

| | |
|---|---|
| Mes, Louis G. B., MD | 1977 |
| Newman, M. Haskell, MD | 1977 |
| Olesen, R. Merrel, MD | 1977 |
| Austad, Eric, MD | 1978 |
| Dempsey, Paul, MD | 1978 |
| Izenberg, Paul, MD | 1978 |
| Argenta, Lou, MD | 1979 |
| Berkowitz, R. Laurence, MD | 1979 |
| Zelnik, Jonathan, MD | 1979 |
| Chapin, Donald, MD | 1980 |
| Gunter, Jack P., MD | 1980 |
| Jones, Neil F., MD | 1981 |
| Manders, Ernest, MD | 1981 |
| Watanabe, Michael, MD | 1981 |
| Gilman, Robert H., MD, DMD | 1982 |
| Fairbanks, Grant, MD | 1982 |
| Harder, Glenn, MD | 1982 |
| Marks, Malcolm, MD | 1982 |

**Reed O. Dingman, MD, DDS, Acting Section Head**

| | |
|---|---|
| Derman, Gordon, MD | 1983 |
| Duus, Erlan, MD | 1983 |
| Friedman, Roger, MD | 1984 |
| Pollock, Richard, MD | 1984 |
| Zucker, Stephen, MD | 1984 |

**Steve Mathes, MD, Section Head**

| | |
|---|---|
| Anderson, Richard, MD | 1985 |
| Hamm, Jeffrey, MD | 1985 |
| Rohrich, Rodney J., MD | 1985 |

*(Continued)*

## 152 Appendix

(Continued)

**Louis Argenta, MD, Section Head**

| | |
|---|---|
| Adson, Martin, MD | 1986 |
| Thornton, James, MD | 1986 |
| VanderKolk, Craig A., MD | 1986 |
| Fang, Kim, MD, DDS | 1987 |
| Iacobucci, John, MD | 1987 |
| Nguyen, Abram, MD | 1987 |

## A-3. Henry Ford Hospital (HFH) and Rotations of Its Residents in Ann Arbor

Drs. Robert Clifford and Alexander Kelly started practice at HFH in Detroit, Michigan, in 1952 and began the residency program there in 1958. Dr. Clifford was the initial chief but died soon thereafter, and Dr. Kelly became chief. Dr. Kelly remained in this position until 1981, when Dr. Don Ditmars, who had rotated in the plastic surgery program in Ann Arbor during his residency at Ford Hospital, became program director. Dr. Robert Pool, one of the early resident trainees at Ford, later started the plastic surgery residency program at William Beaumont Hospital, Royal Oak, Michigan. He innovated an important modification of the Millard unilateral cleft lip repair (previously discussed). As mentioned, he also graciously participated in the teaching program at the University of Michigan over a number of years. According to Dr. John Markley, his father, also a surgeon, knew Dr. Pool at Beaumont and told John that Dr. Pool was also a very proficient hand surgeon. He once presented John with a collection of slides of a very nicely documented series of hand dissections.

### List of HFH Resident Rotators

1962: Cesar Olivas Lozoya, MD
1965: Joe Fox, MD
1966: Earl Norling, MD; Alfred Speirs, MD; and Harvey Weiss, MD
1967: Bob Woodall, MD, and Chosen Lau, MD
1969: Reza Karimipour, MD
1970: Don Ditmars, MD and John Elmquist, MD
1971: John Balfour, MD
1972: W. Peter McCabe, MD
1973: V. Sathyvy, MD
1974: Saleem Malik, MD
1975: Tom Shinabeck, MD
1976: Jorge Gomez, MD
1977: Andrew Abrams, MD

## A-4. Visiting Fellows in the Plastic Surgery Program

1963: G. W. Naraywa SJMH Fellowship
1971: David Chiu-Hwa Lin from Taiwan
1973: Warwick Molteno Montague Morris from South Africa
1973: Samuel Valia
1974: Alphonse Roy from Montreal
1977: Issac Peled from Israel
1978: Khalil Abu-Dalu from Israel
1979: Hassan Badran from Egypt
1981: Paul Tomljanovich from New York City
1982: Georgio Zadini from Italy (stayed only three to four months)

## A-5. Drs. Dingman (ROD), Grabb (WCG), and Oneal's (RMO) Travel Club Members

**Dr. Dingman:** Drs. Joseph Murray, Peter Randall, John M. Converse, Herb Conway, "Willy White," Ralph Millard, Frank Ashley, Paul "Pick" Pickering—met at national meetings and at other times and locations but records not obtainable.

**Dr. Grabb:** Drs. Jerry Bains, Jack Hoopes, Ian Jackson, Josh Jurkiewicz, J. B. Lynch (deceased), Gene Sherlock, John Simons, Jim Smith (deceased), Mel Spira, Hugh Thompson (deceased), Paul Weeks—some of the most prominent men in the field. The meetings always included wives and were held in the host's city and were primarily scientific in content.

**Dr. Oneal:** Drs. Bob Knode, Lenny Glass, Carl Berner, Dave Dingman, Ted Dodenhoff—members were all, except Dave Dingman (who trained with Dr. Ray Broadbent at University of Utah), residents who trained at Michigan in my early years as assistant professor. So we were all close to the same age. All of us had successful private practices in the West and Midwest of the country. All the meetings we had were stag except for one. We always went to some interesting and exciting locale, for skiing, golf, boating, or fishing. About half the time away was spent in formal scientific meetings or informal discussions about techniques, experiences in practice, and unsolved clinical problems.

As different as the groups were, the results were similar in that there was a great deal of interesting, important, and innovative information exchanged, providing a quality of knowledge that is priceless.

154  *Appendix*

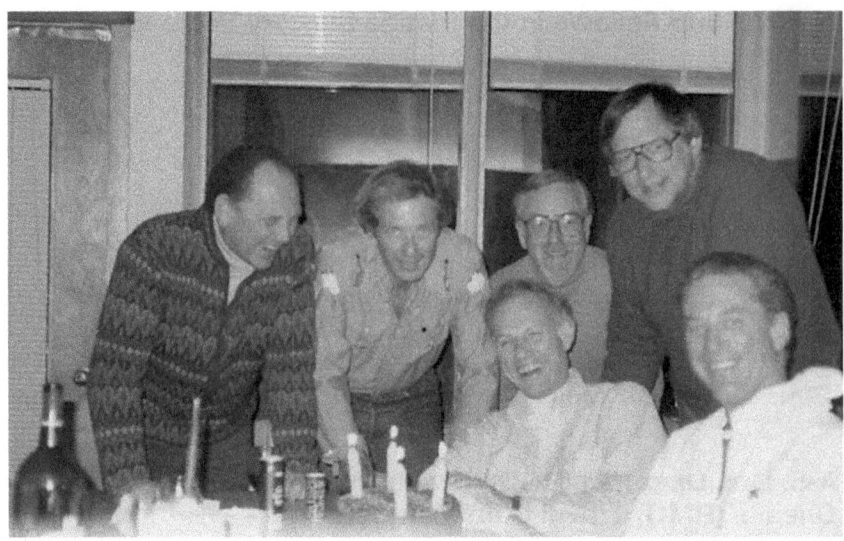

*Photo A5:* Dr. Oneal's travel club.

## A-6. Sasaki's Drawing of Lauralee Lutz

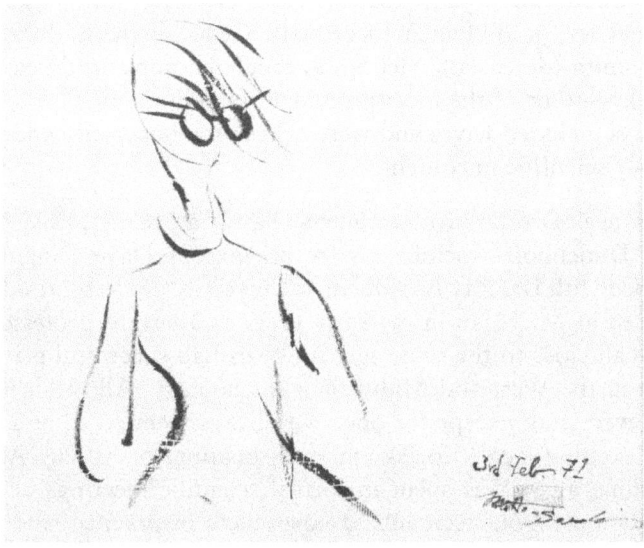

*Photo A6:* Caricature drawn on a napkin by Dr. Moto Sasaki of the Tokyo Police Department. In 1971, he was a visiting professor of plastic surgery at the University of Michigan. Lauralee was a guest at dinner at the Dingmans' together with Dr. Sasaki. After dinner, Dr. Sasaki, also an artist, painted Lauralee's image on a paper napkin as there was no other drawing material available.

## A-7. L3's Remarks about Sasaki's Drawing

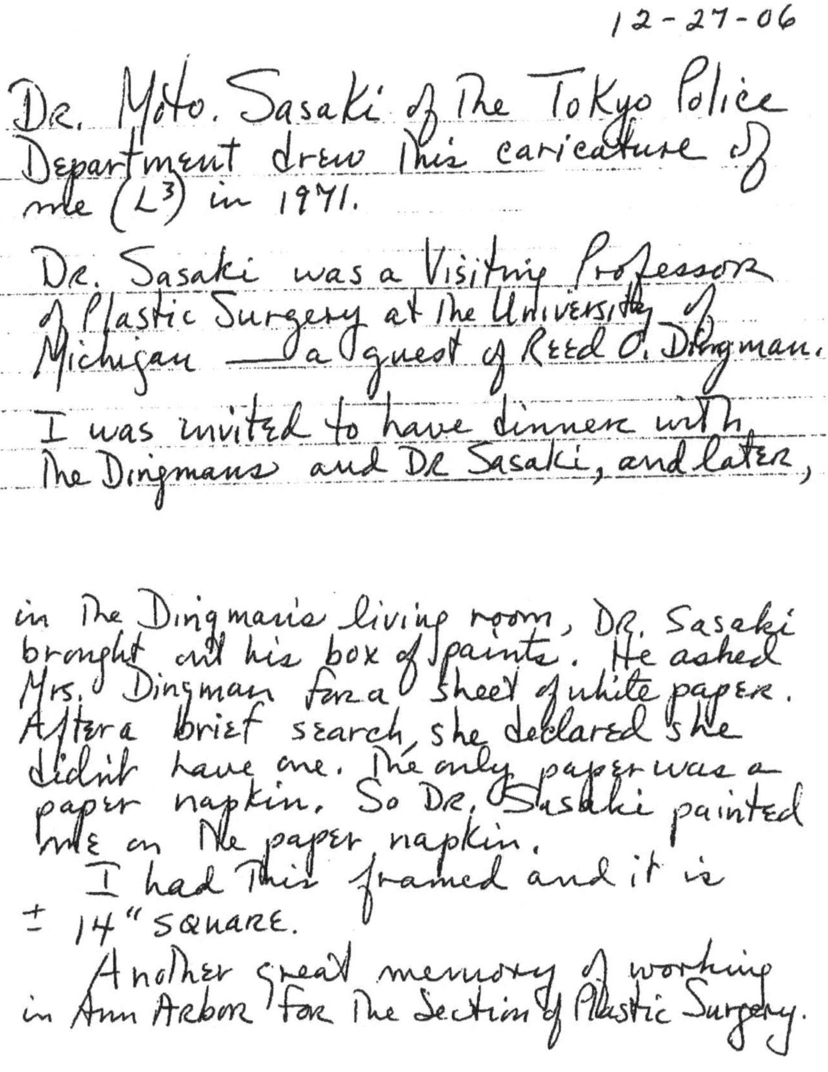

12-27-06

Dr. Moto. Sasaki of The Tokyo Police Department drew this caricature of me (L³) in 1971.

Dr. Sasaki was a Visiting Professor of Plastic Surgery at the University of Michigan — a guest of Reed O. Dingman. I was invited to have dinner with The Dingmans and Dr. Sasaki, and later,

in The Dingman's living room, Dr. Sasaki brought out his box of paints. He asked Mrs. Dingman for a sheet of white paper. After a brief search, she declared she didn't have one. The only paper was a paper napkin. So Dr. Sasaki painted me on the paper napkin.
I had this framed and it is ± 14" square.
Another great memory of working in Ann Arbor for the Section of Plastic Surgery.

*Photo A7:* Lauralee's remarks about Sasaki's drawing.

## A-8. Dr. Grabb's "Ten Most Wanted" Lists

August 13, 1973

TEN MOST WANTED LIST
**********
( A List for Residents of Articles They May Have Missed)

1. Converse, J.M. and Smith, B.: Naso-orbital fractures and traumatic deformities of the medial canthus. Plast. & Reconstr. Surg. 38:147,1966.

2. Millard, D.R.: Closure of bilateral cleft lip and elongation of columella by two operations in infancy. Plast. & Reconstr. Surg. 47:324, 1971.

   Millard, D.R.: Hemirhinoplasty. Plast. & Reconstr. Surg. 40:440, 1967.

3. Goulian, D. and Conway, H.: Prevention of persistent deformity of tragus and lobule by modification of Luckett technique of otoplasty. Plast. & Reconstr. Surg. 26:399, 1960.

4. Daniel, R. and Williams, H.B.: The free transfer of skin flaps by microvascular anastomoses. Plast. & Reconstr. Surg. 52:16, 1973.

5. Stenstrom, S. and Oberg, T.: The nasal deformity in unilateral cleft lip. Plast. & Reconstr. Surg. 28:295, 1961.

6. Thomson, H.G. et al: Surgical tattooing, an experimental study. Plast.& Surg. 37:536, 1966, and Part 2, Plast. & Reconstr. Surg. 39:291, 1967.

7. Niklison, J.: Contribution to the subject of facial paralysis. Plast. & Reconstr. Surg. 17:276, 1956.

8. Luck,J. V.: Dupuytren's contracture; a new concept of the pathogenesis correlated with surgical management. J. Bone & Joint Surg., 41A:635, 1959.

9. Lyons, Chalmers,J.Club (Members-J. Hayward).: Fractures involving mandibular condyles; post treatment survey of 120 cases. J. Oral Surg. 5:45,1947. (This is also on Page 162 of Kazanjian and Converse's book on <u>Surgical Treatment of Facial Injuries.</u>)

10. Tsuge,K.: Treatment of macrodactyly. Plast. & Reconstr. Surg. 39:590,1967.

BONUS-
Bunnell, S.: Atraumatic technique. Calif. State J. Med. 19:204, 1921.
(This also appears in Bunnell's <u>Surgery of the Hand</u>, 3rd Edition, 1956,p.105).

Read everything written by Dingman, Millard, Stenstrom, and Converse.

-W.C. Grabb

*Photo A8:* As Dr. Grabb kindly stated, these are "lists for the residents of articles they may have missed." The first list appeared in August 1973, followed by a second one in November. We all appreciated his persistent and helpful efforts to keep us informed.

November 19, 1973

***** 2$^{nd}$ TEN MOST WANTED LIST *****

(Some pearls that may have escaped you ...)

1. Simon, B.E., Hoffman, S., and Kahn, S.: Classification and surgical correction of gynecomastia. Plast. & Reconstr. Surg. 51,48, 1973.

2. Leake, D., Doykos, J., Habal, M., and Murray, J.E.: Long-term follow-up of fractures of the mandibular condyle in children. Plast. & Reconstr. Surg. 47:127, 1971.

3. Millard, D.R.:Alar margin sculpturing. Plast. & Reconstr. Surg. 40:337, 1967.

4. Knowles, C.C.: Changes in the profile following surgical reduction of mandibular prognathism. Brit. J. Plast. Surg. 18:432, 1965.

5. Crikelair, G.F. and Cosman, B.: Histologically benign, clinically malignant lesions of head and neck. Plast. & Reconstr. Surg. 42:343, 1968.

6. Musgrave, R.H.: Variations on the correction of congenital lop ear. Plast. & Reconstr. Surg. 37:394, 1966.

7. Edgerton, M.T.: Surgical lengthening of external nose to correct congenital or traumatic arrest of nasal growth. Plast. & Reconstr. Surg. 38:320, 1966.

8. Crawford, B.S., and Vivakanathan, C: The treatment of giant cystic hygroma of the neck. Brit. J. Plast. Surg. 26:69, 1973.

9. Loeb, R.: Technique for preservation of the temporal branches of the facial nerve during face-left operation. Brit. J. Plast. Surg. 23:390, 1970.

10. Argamaso, R.V. and Lewin, M.: Repair of partial ear loss with local composite flaps. Plast. & Reconstr. Surg. 42:437, 1968.

******

*Photo A8:* (Continued)

158 *Appendix*

## A-9. Two Letters Regarding Changes in ROD Society

*221 North Ingalls / Ann Arbor, Michigan 48104 / Area Code 313—761-7920*

REED O. DINGMAN, M. D. *Plastic Surgery*

23 March 1981

William C. Grabb, M.D.
C7200 Outpatient, Box 22
University Hospital
Ann Arbor, MI 48109

Dear Bill:

As you must know, I was pleased and highly honored when the society representing the trainees of the Plastic Surgery Service at the University of Michigan formed the Reed O. Dingman Society in 1963, through the efforts of Paul Natvig, Clyde Litton and you. The Society has grown and prospered and now comprises a large membership. Up until this time, it has been a largely social group, bound together by the commonality of having trained at the University of Michigan. Its informality has been one of its charms. However, many significant changes have occurred since the founding of the Society in 1963.

It occurs to me that the Society might serve a more purposeful function in teaching research and dissemination of knowledge in our chosen field by a more formal organizational structure, and defining its future objectives. In your position of leadership, you are naturally the one that would be most influential in bringing about some changes that would directly benefit the training program at the University of Michigan Hospital.

I should be pleased to discuss this with you further at your convenience Last October at the Meeting of the American Society of Plastic and Reco: structive Surgeons in New Orleans, I was elected as the first honorary member of the D. Ralph Millard Plastic Surgical Society. It was an impressive experience and was the stimulus that initiated this letter to you. The enclosure may be of interest to you and give you some ideas.

Sincerely,

Reed O. Dingman, M.D.
Enclosure
ROD:law

---

*Photo A9:* The first letter is from March 23, 1981, from Dr. Dingman to Dr. Grabb, asking him to consider facilitating some changes to the ROD Society to promote teaching, research, and knowledge dissemination. The second is from Dr. Grabb to Lenny Glass (resident, 1968–70), asking Glass to head a committee to spell out the process of making these changes.

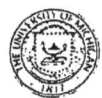

WILLIAM C. GRABB, M.D.
Plastic & Reconstructive Surgery

November 9, 1981

Leonard W. Glass, M.D.
255 N. Elm Street
Escondido, California 02025

Dear Lennie:

    Here I am again calling upon you to help.

    It is becoming increasingly apparent to me that there is a desire that the Reed O. Dingman Society serve a more purposeful function. Enclosed is information from Reed Dingman, as well as Bob Wilensky regarding this.

    I would like this Committee to be headed by you and consist of Bob Oneal, Bob Wilensky, and two others of your choosing. I would ask that you correspond, and probably eventually hold a conference call, to discuss the directions that the Reed O. Dingman Society should take. I would further ask that you contact Richard Greminger regarding details on how the Millard Society functions, and possibly Peter Randall regarding the University of Pennsylvania Society and Joe McCarthy regarding the New York University Society.

    My personal wish is that this new direction will involve the support of our Plastic Surgery Research Program, such as you are familiar with through the Plastic Surgery Research Advisory Committee.

    Reed has again this week expressed his wishes that such directions be undertaken. I would like to see that you and your Committee follow through.

    With best regards.

                                     Very truly yours,

                                     Bill

                                   William C. Grabb, M.D.
                                   Professor of Surgery & Head,
                                   Section of Plastic Surgery

WCG/acv
enclosures

*Photo A9:* (Continued)

## A-10. Eulogy for Dr. William C. Grabb by Dr. Oneal

IN MEMORIUM

WILLIAM C. GRABB, M.D. 1928-1982

I was honored when Cozy asked me to speak at this service in Bill's memory, and it is with love for both Bill and Cozy as well as Betsy, David, and Anne that I consented to say a few words.

Bill Grabb was a dear friend for more than 20 years. During the early years of the Section of Plastic Surgery at the University, I was lucky enough to be associated in practice and teaching with Dr. Dingman and Bill. During those years the three of us became like a family, and the central core of a larger family ...many of whom are here today. This feeling of unity continues to nourish us as we struggle to carry on after Bill's death.

I've never had a brother, but I think that that is what Bill Grabb was to me. We sometimes fought and disagreed, but always reconciled and respected each other's opinions. I think we came to love each other. My life is immensely diminished by his death.

We were four years apart in age...just enough so that he had usually completed what I yet dreamed of doing. Bill's accomplishments, which to most of us are only dreams, will always be an inspiration to me. His high standards and expectations have helped me to achieve what I never would have without him.

He was a man of his word. I could count on him to give me a fair hearing. He would incorporate the good ideas of his colleagues into his plans which made us all respect him as a leader.

Bill was generous in sharing with me the world of plastic surgery that he had helped Dr. Dingman create in Ann Arbor. For that I am eternally grateful.

When sorting out my feelings during the past two weeks, I remembered a quotation from William Penn which Bill had written on the flyleaf of the copy of the first edition of his plastic surgery textbook when he gave it to me. I would like to share it with you today:

"The Friendship between me and you I will not compare to a chain -- for that might rust or a falling tree might break."

This feeling of an everlasting bond between friends and loved ones is what Bill believed in. It is what links all of us who were fortunate enough to have our lives touched by him. It is what links all of us to Bill Grabb's spirit into Eternity.

-Robert Moore Oneal, M.D.
Sunday, April 4, 1982
First Presbyterian Church of Ann Arbor

*Photo A10:* The eulogy I gave at Bill Grabb's memorial service in 1982 at the First Presbyterian Church, Ann Arbor, Michigan.

## A-11. Memorial Remarks from the Final Group of Residents Who Trained under Dr. Grabb

Memorial Remarks from His Residents

WILLIAM C. GRABB, M.D. 1928-1982

As the last group of residents to be trained by Dr. Grabb at the University of Michigan, we are acutely aware of his passing. We wish to express not only our enormous sadness over his loss, but also our gratitude for what he meant to us as a teacher and friend.

Dr. Grabb created for all of us in the residency program a unique atmosphere for academic pursuits that was stimulating, challenging and pleasurable. His great talent for teaching set an example in humility and honesty which will always remain dear to us.

We offer our deepest regrets to his beloved wife, Cozette, and his family, and feel extremely honored to have had the privilege of studying with such a kind and knowledgeable man.

>Gordon H. Derman, M.D.
>Erlan C. Duus, M.D.
>Roger J. Friedman, M.D.
>Robert H. Gilman, M.D., D.M.D.
>Glenn C. Harder, M.D.
>Malcolm W. Marks, M.D.

Ann Arbor, Michigan

April 8, 1982

*Photo A11:* The memorial remarks were later published in the *Plastic and Reconstructive Surgery* journal and accompanied the eulogy for Dr. Grabb by Dr. Dingman that has been quoted in the main text.

## A-12. The Cover of the Book *A Message to Garcia*

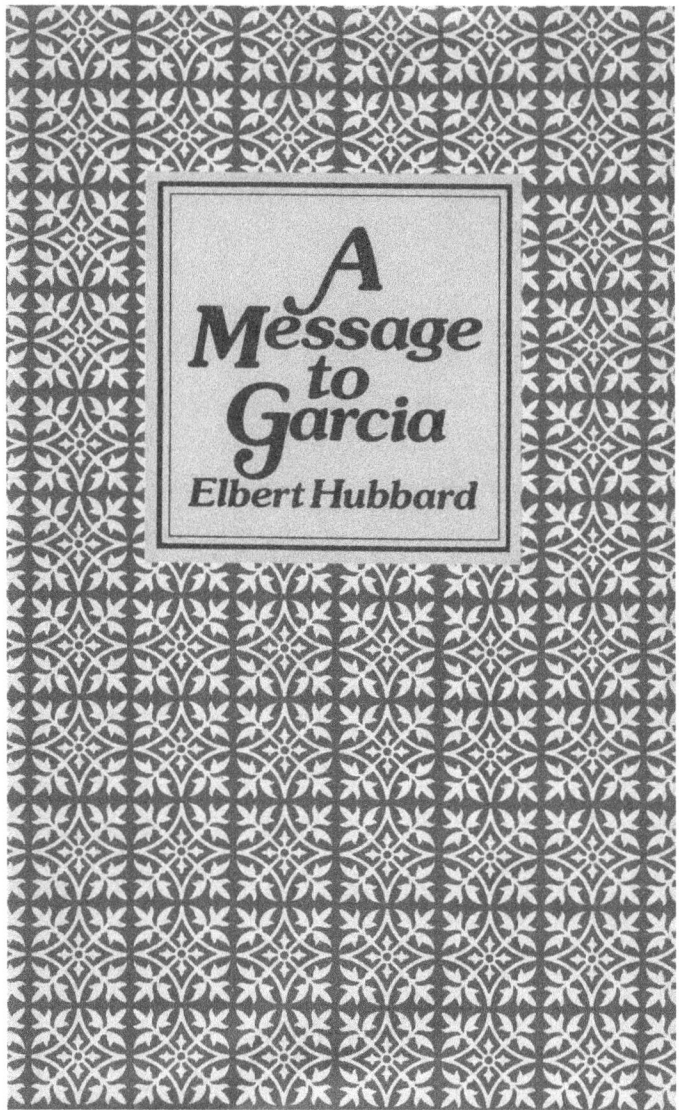

*Photo A12:* The book tells the story of a young lieutenant in the US Army, Andrew Rowan, during the Spanish-American War. He was sent on a mission to find the leader of the Cuban revolution and deliver a message from President McKinley. He landed alone and in secret in Cuba. Under harsh and dangerous circumstances, he successfully delivered the important message to General Garcia, who was in charge of the Revolutionary forces. Bill Grabb deeply respected the courage and spirit in "delivering the message" and "finishing the job."[1]

## A-13. Letter from Lauralee Lutz to Dr. Dingman

REED O. DINGMAN, M.D.
Plastic & Reconstructive Surgery

August 29, 1983

Reed O. Dingman, M.D., F.A.C.S.
Professor of Surgery & Acting Head,
Section of Plastic Surgery

Dear Dr. Dingman:

More than anyone else around here YOU deserve a letter of thanks from all of us for gluing us together and maintaining the leadership necessary to get us through our dark days and back into the sunshine of the future.

I can only imagine the extent of your personal sacrifice in returning to the University, just when you and Mrs. Dingman thought you could travel or do other enjoyable things together. The adjustment has been enormous for both of you, and we should never have asked it, but in fact you have delivered more than anyone could have dreamed. You bring 52 years of medical experience to our Section, along with a lifetime of very special human skills in understanding people. You teach all of us how to be consistently kind, thoughtful, polite, clean, and duty-bound. No one teaches such values any more in school, but you teach every day by example.

I have always been honored and proud to be associated with you, and still worry a little about seeing things from your point of view so I can represent you and do things the way you would choose to have them done. I want to be perfect to fit in with your accomplishments. My promise to you for the coming academic year is that I will keep trying, and as a team we will do whatever needs to be done.

Sincerely,

Lauralee A. Lutz
Your Secretary

lal

C7200 Outpatient Building/University Hospital/Ann Arbor, Michigan 48109/313-764-3290

*Photo A13:* Letter from Lauralee to Dr. Dingman expressing her gratitude and her unqualified support for him after he assumed the leadership of the Section of Plastic Surgery following Dr. Grabb's death.

## A-14. Quotes from William Osler

221 North Ingalls / Ann Arbor, Michigan 48104 / Area Code 313—761-7920

REED O. DINGMAN, M. D. *Plastic Surgery*

January 11, 1979

Miss Laura Lee Lutz
Section of Plastic Surgery
7th Level - Outpatient Building
University Hospital
Ann Arbor, MI  48109

Dear Laura Lee,

The following two quotations are by Dr. William Osler from his book entitled "Books and Men."

"For the teacher and student [*the worker*] a great library such as this is indispensable. They must know the world's best work and know it at once."

Perhaps he is better known for the following:

"To study the phenomena of disease without books is to sail an uncharted sea, while to study books without patients is not to go to sea at all."

It would be very fitting, I think, to have these printed by the Medical Art people and have them framed and hung in the Reed O. Dingman library.

Here's another one:

"It is in utilizing the fresh knowledge of the journals that the young physician may attain quickly the name and fame he desires."  Sir William Osler.

Sincerely,

Reed O. Dingman, M.D.

ROD/dls

+ *A good surgeon should always be his own severest critic* — Milton Adams

---

*Photo A14:* Quotes that Dr. Dingman proposed be framed and hung in the Reed O. Dingman Library on the sixth floor of the outpatient building at the university hospital. Also included were additional quotations from Milton Adams, Cicero, Samuel Butler, Longfellow, and Donne, and one additional quote from Dr. Grabb.

A friend, one might say, a second self.

                Cicero

Going away.
I can generally bear the separation, but I don't like the leave-taking.

                Samuel Butler

Lives of great men all remind us
We can make our lives sublime,
And, departing, leave behind us
Footprints in the sands of time.

                Longfellow

No man is an island, entire of itself;
Every man is a piece of the continent...;
Any man's death diminishes me, because
I am involved in mankind.

                Donne

I will forever thank the unseen forces that caused our paths to cross and then head out in the same direction.

                W.C.Grabb

*Photo A14:* (Continued)

# A-15. A Copy of Dr. Dingman's Motto, Quotations, and Advice to Residents

DR. REED O. DINGMAN

Motto:     You are what you are.
           You must what you must.
           It costs what it costs.        -Author unknown.

Favorite Quotations:

"A teacher affects eternity; he can never tell where his influence stops." - Henry Adams

"To study the phenomena of disease without books is to sail an uncharted sea, while to study books without patients is not to go to sea at all." -Sir William Osler

Advice to Residents:

Always make the most of your experience, no matter how tedious. You can always learn something from every case you do. Your duty is to render the best possible care to all our patients. Be prompt, helpful, and courteous...show your interest...

You can always learn something from every case if you wish to. Or you can complain and annoy yourself and all of those around you if that is what you choose. I can only assure you that the former course is the wiser.

Keep all of your relationships cordial. If incidents arise ...usually problems can be resolved in an amicable fashion in high level discussion.

*Photo A15.* A copy of Dr. Dingman's motto, two favorite quotations, one by Osler mentioned in A-14 and the other by Henry Adams, who was a historian and a great grandson to President John Adams and grandson of President John Quincy Adams. Also included is Dr. Dingman's advice to residents as remembered by Lauralee. In addition is a mention as to what he felt was his greatest honor and a statement as to how proud he was of his trainees.

Dr. Dingman-11/3/83

The Greatest Honor:

"The responsibility of serving on the Accreditation and Certification Board of one's chosen specialty is the greatest honor that can come to any doctor."

ROD as Chairman of the American Board of Plastic Surgery - 1965

On Residents:

"We are proud of all our boys, aren't we? (to L-3)."

Referring to @70 graduates of the U-M residency program

*Photo A15.* (Continued)

## A-16. Gillies's Painting

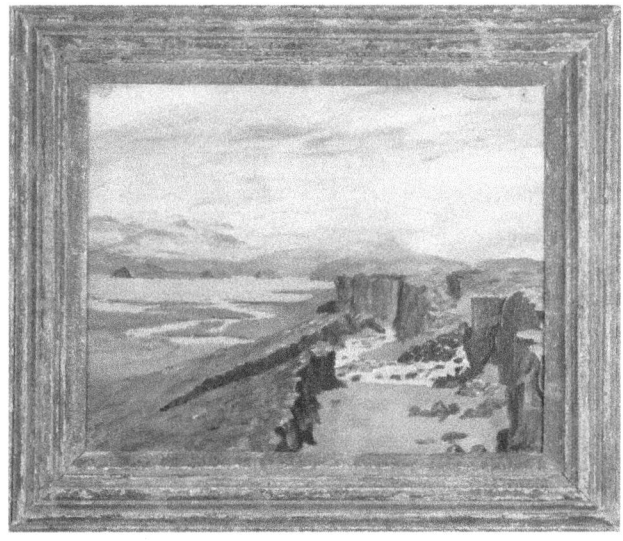

*Photo A16:* The painting, "The Great Rift," by Sir Harold Gillies, depicts "rift" or separation in Iceland between the American and Eurasian tectonic plates. It is also the geographic location of several historical events in Iceland. The fascinating journey of this painting was related to me by Sigurdur (Siggi) Thorvaldsson (resident, 1971–73). Siggi first saw the painting hanging in Dr. Dingman's private office when he arrived for a resident interview in 1969. Apparently, Dr. Ralph Millard had received the painting as a gift from Gillies following the collaboration on the book, *Principles and Art of Plastic Surgery*. At a later date, Millard gave it to his close friend Reed O. Dingman. Following Dr. Dingman's death in 1985, the painting came to the possession of his son David. He subsequently sent it to Siggi who now has it hanging in his home in Reykjavik, Iceland. This saga was published in the *Annals of Plastic Surgery*.[2]

## A-17. Lauralee's Eulogy Letter for Dr. Dingman in 1985

REED O. DINGMAN, M.D.
1906-1985

The tallest, straightest, most perfect tree dominating the forest is often called the Witness Tree. This is because it has personal knowledge of the rest of the forest by benefit of its age and height. It has been there the longest and seen the most. Nothing escapes its notice. The tread of a squirrel, fall of the leaves, storms and seasons are all witnessed. It is exemplary and protective.

Some men become Witness Trees to their profession. They achieve more, contribute more, set a higher example, and attract a larger group of people to influence. They become the guide, the inspiration, and the caretaker of those coming up alongside.

Reed O. Dingman was a Witness Tree in American plastic and reconstructive surgery for over 50 years.

His presence in any group, large or small, local, national or international, was an inspiration of leadership and guidance. He led young developing physicians and surgeons along a well marked path yet allowed for strays and reconnoitering. He listened as much as he talked. He learned from everyone and was astonished when this trait was not the denominator throughout professional circles.

He was wise.
He was sensible and kind.

He understood that life is a matter of sequences and consequences.
He noticed the world around him and pronounced it "good."
He was a happy man.

He was dignified. He did not need the shallow frenzy of haste, noise, or a display of temper to announce his arrival or to intimidate others. He always had time to be polite.

***

Dr. Dingman was a giant in our land, and now he is of the land. But he can still be our Witness Tree, guiding and inspiring us to grow and reach to the height of our abilities.

If we keep him in our hearts he will still help us. Just as he did all along.

Lauralee A. Lutz
Ann Arbor, Michigan
December 1985

*Photo A17:* Lauralee's eulogy and remembrances sent to all members of the ROD Society following Dr. Dingman's death on December 24, 1985.

## A-18. Eulogy by David L. Dingman, MD, for His Father

```
            REED O. DINGMAN, M.D.
                 1906-1985
```

Reed Dingman died on December 24th at 4:15 p.m.
We gather here in this small group, limited in numbers, as he would have wished. It is characteristic that he wished to be attended by a few close relatives and friends to avoid inconveniencing others during the Christmas holiday.

I attended him at death as he attended me at birth, thus completing the circle. He died as he had lived, with dignity.

His accomplishments have been widely chronicled and we of his inner circle need not repeat them now. Physically, intellectually, and emotionally he was the finest man I knew, but I would rather dwell in another area.

All of us here shared in his most marvelous quality; the sincere ability to reach into every person and find the best. The bonding that this produced allowed us to join him in the celebration of life. A life that always seemed to have perfect balance between hard work, ample reward, and subtle reflection.

He moved through life with the calmness of a perfectly trimmed sailing ship. He gathered his crew from those adrift in a confused sea, leaving smoothness in his wake. Those who elected to sail a different course did so with his blessing, and remained lifelong friends. He encountered obstacles and heavy weather but he seemed to have the magical quality to turn problems into

*Photo A18.* Eulogy by David L. Dingman for Reed O. Dingman at his funeral service in Ann Arbor on December 27, 1985.

Page 2-Dr. Reed O. Dingman

opportunities and foes into friends and co-workers. He is silent now and we must sail on alone, but the course is clear because we have traveled with the master.

He was proudest of his role as a teacher but even he could not appreciate the breadth of the subjects he taught. Here was a man who lived life as it ought to be lived, a perfect role model not only as a physician but as a man at peace with the world, and this is his greatest legacy.

We must do our grieving but let us soon turn to joyous remembrances of how he enriched our lives.

                                                David L. Dingman, M.D.
                                                December 27, 1985
                                                Ann Arbor, Michigan

*Photo A18.* (Continued)

## A-19. Eulogy by Dr. Oneal

REED O. DINGMAN, M.D.
1906-1985

Reed O. Dingman was born on November 4, 1906 in Rockwood, Michigan and died after a short illness on December 24, 1985. He is survived by his wife, Thelma, and his children Sue, Sally and David, as well as 12 grandchildren.

Dr. Dingman graduated from the University of Michigan Dental School in 1931 and received his Masters in Science and Oral Surgery in 1932. He then graduated from the University of Michigan Medical School in 1936. He continued the practice of oral surgery while pursuing additional training in maxillofacial surgery during 1936-1939, and in plastic surgery from 1945-1946. At that time he began his practice of plastic surgery at St. Joseph Mercy Hospital in Ann Arbor, with his office at 221 North Ingalls Street, across the street from the hospital. He single handedly established plastic and reconstructive surgery as an important and well respected specialty in Ann Arbor. His practice became an international center with a constant stream of national and internationally renowned plastic surgery visitors and fellows as his reputation spread.

He was the author of a major textbook on facial fractures, with one of his earliest trainees, Paul Natvig, and contributed significantly to 24 other major textbooks on plastic and reconstructive surgery. In addition, he wrote 130 articles on a wide range of clinical problems.

During the course of his career, Dr. Dingman received the ultimate esteem of his peers by being elected president of the American Society of Plastic and Reconstructive Surgeons as well as of its Educational Foundation. He was also president of the American Society of Maxillofacial Surgeons and served on the American Board of Plastic Surgery, acting as its Chairman in 1963-1964.

*Photo A19:* Eulogy by Dr. Oneal for Dr. Dingman, read on March 18, 1986, at the Quarterly meeting of the medical staff at SJMH.

Page 2- Obituary -SJMH
      Reed O. Dingman, M.D.

In 1954, with the help and support of Sister Mary Xavier, he founded a plastic surgery residency at St. Joseph Mercy Hospital. This became a center of excellence and was the nucleus of the integrated program with the University of Michigan that followed in 1964. Dr. Dingman became Professor and Head of the Section of Plastic Surgery at the University but continued to maintain a very active practice at St. Joseph Mercy Hospital. Under his influence I think the affiliation of the two institutions has been and remains a model for cooperation and mutual respect right up to the present time.

Those of us who worked closely with him remember his late office hours (until 10:00 or 11:00 at night) as he adjusted the schedule for his teaching commitment while maintaining his practice and activities at this institution. He expected a great deal of all those who worked with him, but no more than he expected of himself.

In 1976 Dr. Dingman retired as the Head of the Section of Plastic Surgery at the University to be succeeded by Bill Grabb. Another measure of his greatness was his ability to remain active and supportive in the teaching program without undermining Bill's authority and leadership. Immediately after Bill's untimely death in 1982, and although he was now 76 years of age, Dr. Dingman graciously accepted the position of Acting Head at the University providing essential leadership and stability at a time of crisis. When a permanent chief was selected in 1984, Dr. Dingman retired again but remained on staff as an active and potent force in the teaching program until his death. His influence was noted by one of our residents who just graduated last July and who wrote upon hearing of Dr. Dingman's death," The opportunity of working with Dr. Dingman was truly a high point in the Ann Arbor experience. He taught all of us so much about patient care and working with people."

This letter emphasized what we all knew about Dr. Dingman's gentleness, compassion, and open-mindedness which was returned by the love and respect of his many thousands of patients throughout the years. These qualities, as

*Photo A19:* (Continued)

Page 3- Obituary-SJMH
Reed O. Dingman,M.D.

much as his great surgical skill and intellectual accomplishments became a role model for three generations of plastic surgical trainees. The formation of the Reed O. Dingman Society in 1961 and its reorganization in 1984 into a scientific as well as social organization is a testament to the respect more than 75 of his trainees hold for him.

I believe that all of us should remember Reed Dingman with gratitude for his long term commitment to the excellence of this hospital and all it stands for. He will be sorely missed, not only by his friends and colleagues, but by all those in our hospital family who came into contact with him in his daily work. We will always remember his warm smile and friendly greetings, and genuine interest in us as people not only as employees.

We of the Medical Staff of St. Joseph Mercy Hospital extend our deepest and most sincere sympathy to Mrs. Dingman and the children in this time of loss.

Robert M. Oneal, M.D.
March 18, 1986

Read at the Catherine McAuley Health Center
Quarterly meeting of the Medical Staff

Photo A19: (Continued)

# Group Images of Residents

Code: RG = resident (plastic surgery senior) graduates, with year graduated in; JR = junior plastic surgery residents; 3&3 = 3&3 residency pathway; OT = other residents; TF = teaching faculty; Flw = fellow; HFR = Henry Ford Rotator; Lab = research lab; NI = not able to identify. All will be identified from left to right in the images. FR = front row; BR = back row. All MDs unless specified.

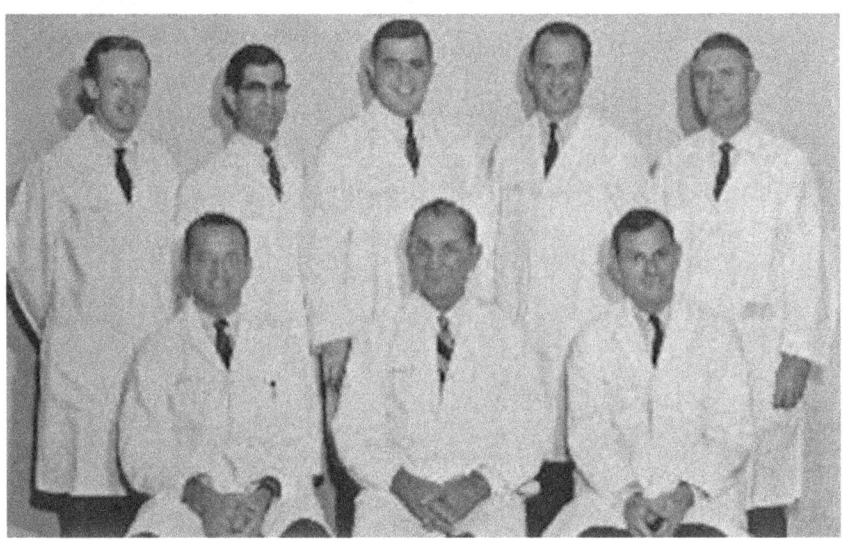

*Photo 1967:*

**FR:** Grabb, Dingman (section head), Oneal (all TF)
**BR:** Chapple, Constant, Wilms (all JR); Knode RG-1967; Russell RG-1967

Leaders in Plastic Surgery 175

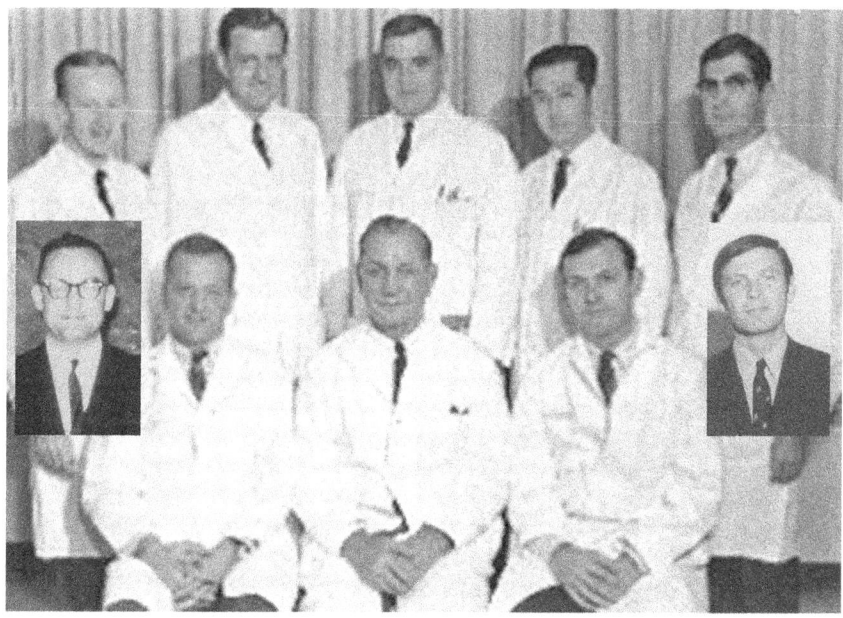

Photo 1968: A composite photograph of RG graduates in 1968 and 1969, with two people added by the authors to make the groups complete.

**FR:** Borocz RG-1969; Grabb, Dingman, Oneal (all TF); Dodenhoff RG-1969
**BR:** Chapple RG-1968, Seaton RG-1969, Wilms RG-1968, Ramos RG-1969, Constant RG-1968

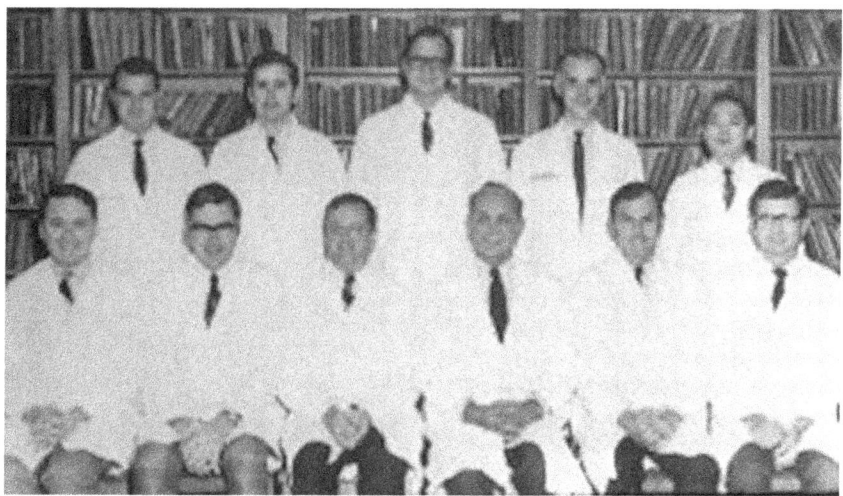

Photo 1970:

**FR:** Glass RG-1970; Hudak RG-1970; Grabb, Dingman, Oneal (all TF); Kloster RG-1970
**BR:** Wersky (left program after one year); Fairbanks, Berner (both JR); Balfour HFR; Lin Flw

## Group Images of Residents

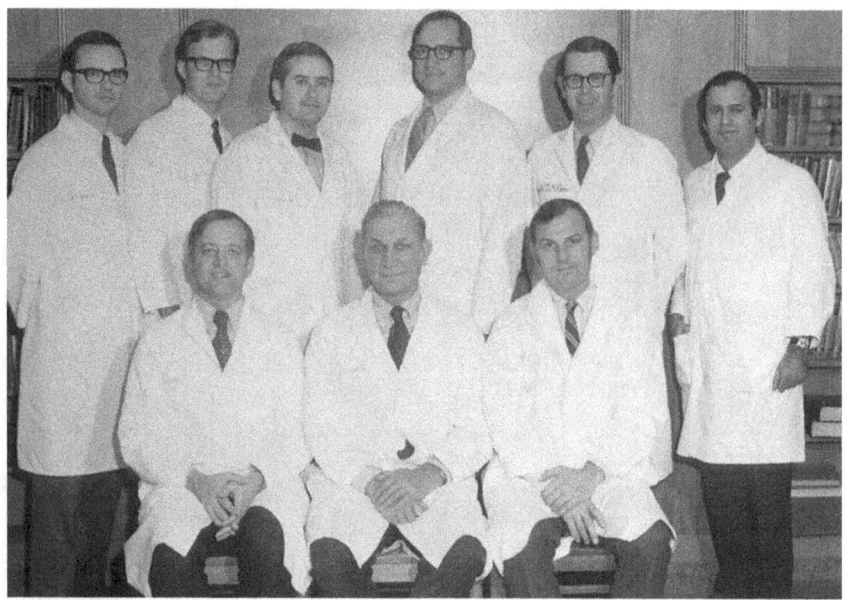

*Photo 1971:*

**FR:** Grabb, Dingman, Oneal (all TF)
**BR:** Greer, Geisterfer (both JR); Fairbanks RG-1971; Berner RG-1971; McCabe HFR; Wexler JR

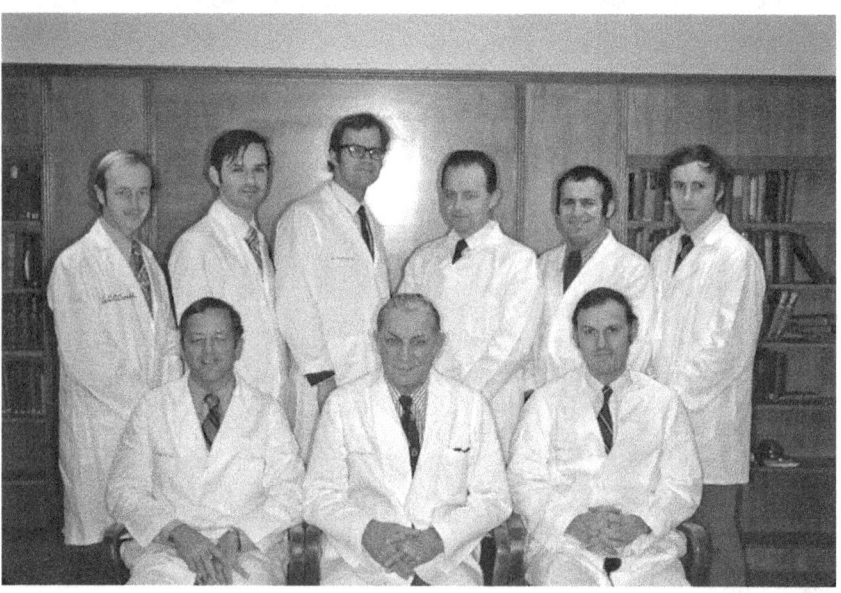

*Photo 1972:*

**FR:** Grabb, Dingman, Oneal (all TF)
**BR:** Cromwell JR, Greer RG-1972, Geisterfer RG-1972, Thorvaldssen JR, Wexler RG-1972, Nobel JR

*Leaders in Plastic Surgery* 177

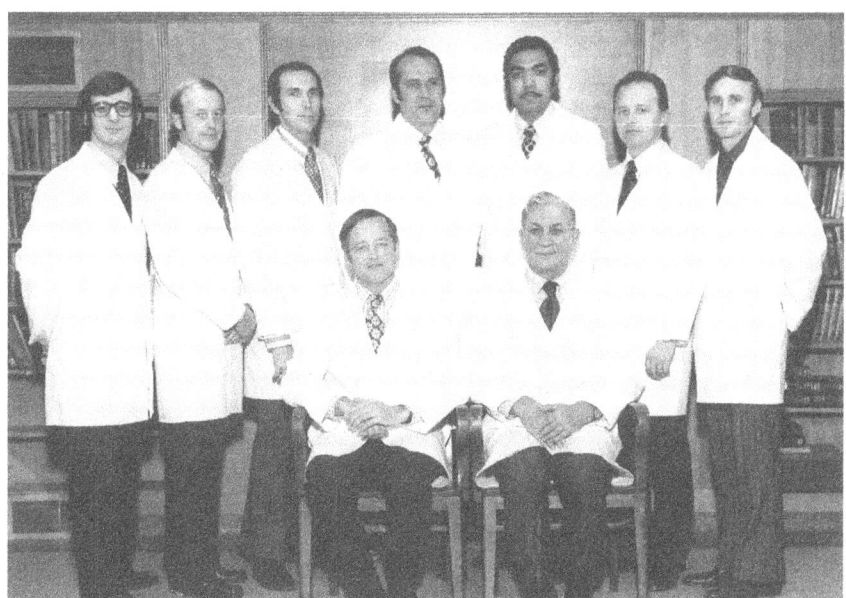

Photo 1973:

**FR:** Grabb, Dingman (both TF)
**BR:** Roy Flw; Cromwell RG-1973; Novak, O'Connor, Norris (all JR); Thorvaldssen RG-1973; Nobel RG-1973

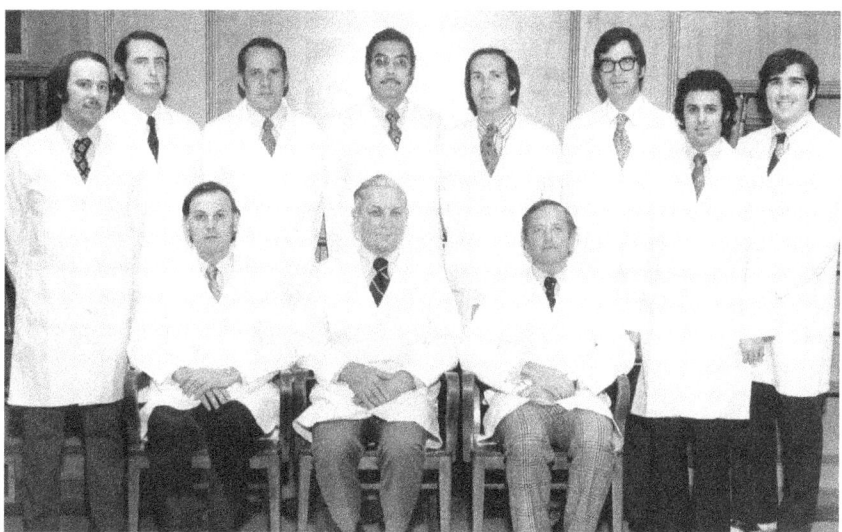

Photo 1974:

**FR:** Oneal, Dingman, Grabb (all TF)
**BR:** Lawrence JR; Morris Flw; O'Conner RG-1974; Norris RG-1974; Novark RG-1974; MacCollum, Wilensky (both JR); Gingrass OT

## 178  Group Images of Residents

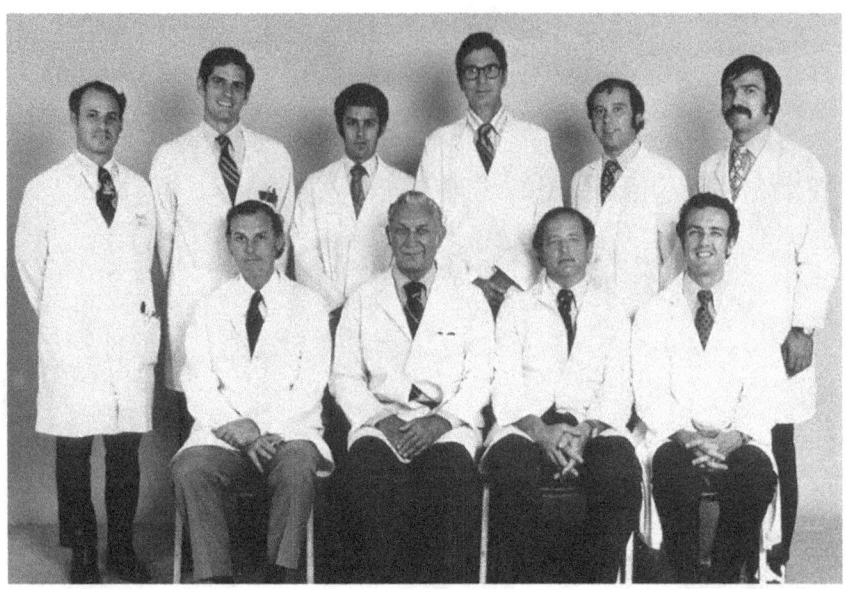

*Photo 1975:*

**FR:** Oneal, Dingman, Grabb, Markley (all TF)
**BR:** Agris, Blackburn (both JR); Wilensky RG-1975; MacCollum RG-1975; Lawrence RG-1975; Bucko JR

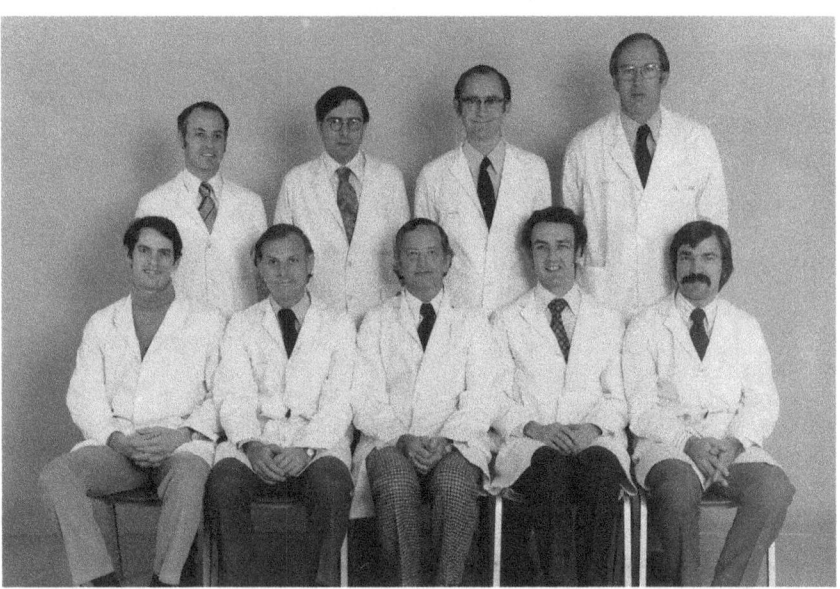

*Photo 1976:*

**FR:** Blackburn RG-1976; Oneal, Grabb (now Section Head), Markley (all TF); Bucko RG-1976
**BR:** Agris RG-1976, Abrams HFR, Mes, Olesen (both JR)

Leaders in Plastic Surgery 179

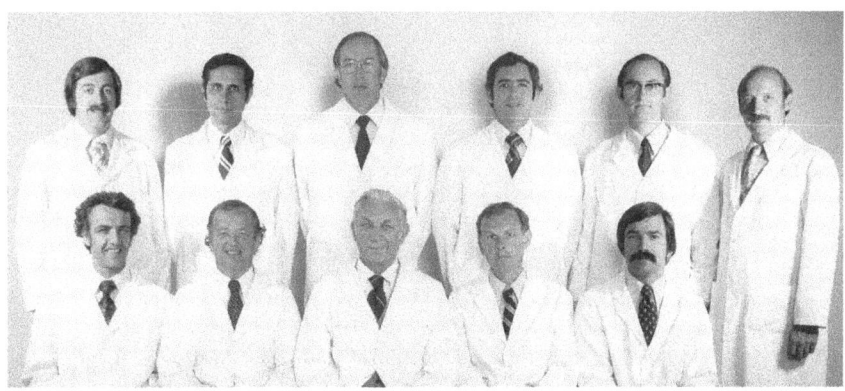

Photo 1977:

**FR:** Markley, Grabb, Dingman, Oneal, Bucko (all TF)
**BR:** Dempsey JR, Badran Flw, Olesen RG-1977, Izenberg JR, Mes RG-1977, Newman RG-1977

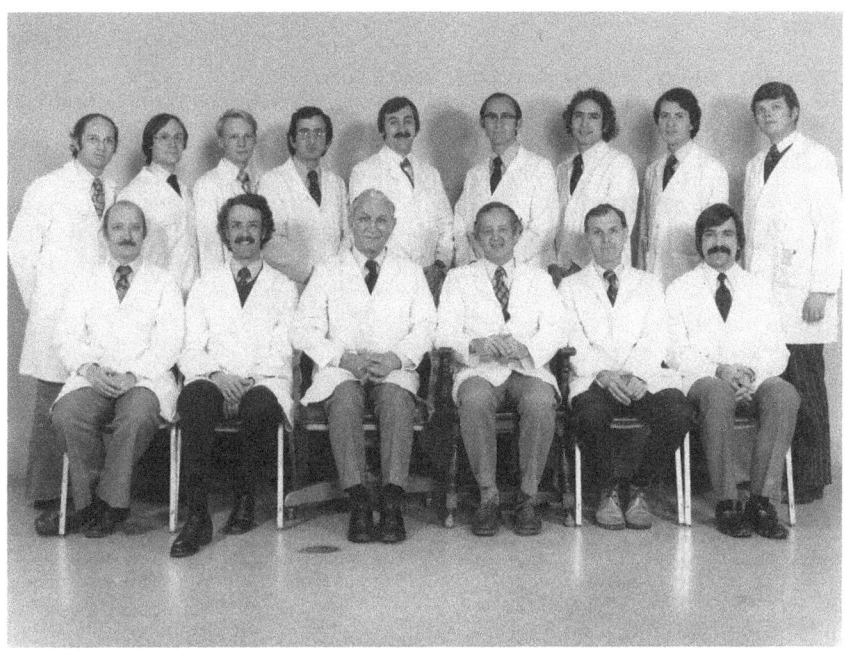

Photo 1978:

**FR:** Newman, Markley, Dingman, Grabb, Oneal, Bucko (all TF)
**BR:** Peled Flw, Berkowitz JR, Harder 3&3, Argenta JR, Dempsey RG-1978, Mes TF, Izenberg RG-1978, Zelnik JR, Austad RG-1978

180   *Group Images of Residents*

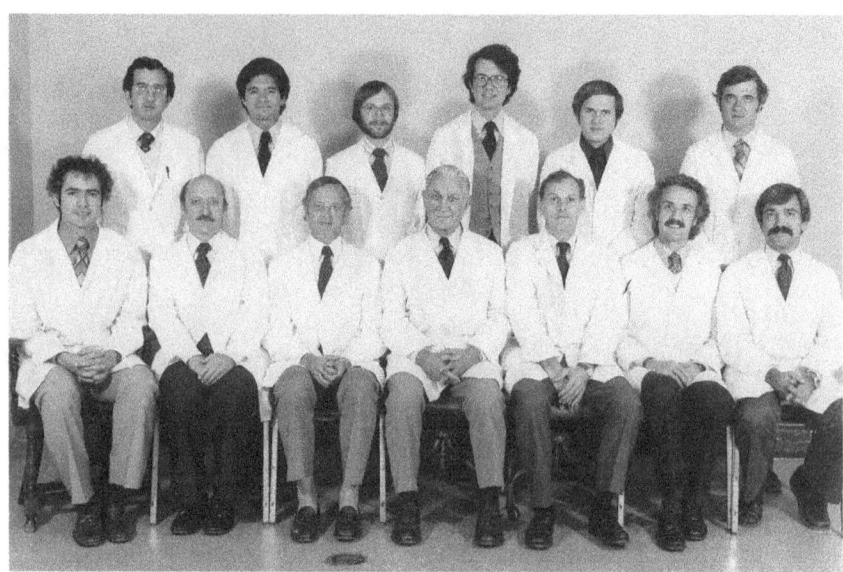

*Photo 1979:*

**FR:** Izenberg, Newman, Grabb, Dingman, Oneal, Markley, Bucko (all TF)
**BR:** Argenta RG-1979, Gemberling (left program), Berkowitz RG-1979, Zelnik RG-1979, Chapin JR, Cherry Lab.

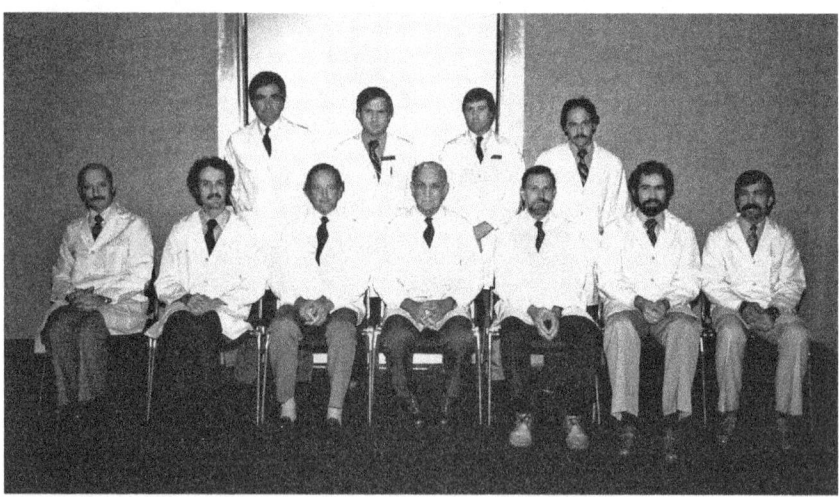

*Photo 1980:*

**FR:** Newman, Markley, Grabb, Dingman, Oneal, Izenberg, Bucko (all TF)
**BR:** Gunter RG-1980, Chapin RG-1980, Jones JR, NI

## Leaders in Plastic Surgery 181

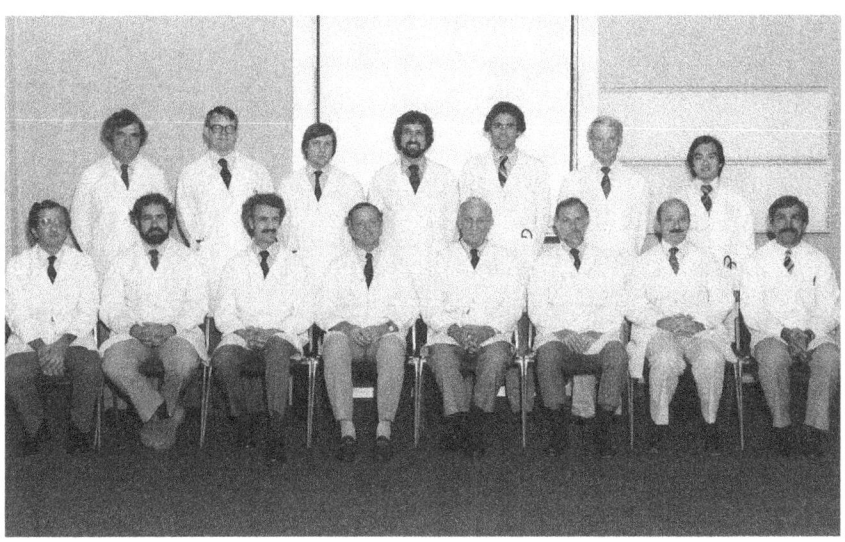

*Photo 1981:*

**FR:** Argenta, Izenberg, Markley, Grabb, Dingman, Oneal, Newman, Bucko (all TF)
**BR:** Cherry Lab; Manders RG-1981; Jones RG-1981; Gilman, Marks, Harder (all JR); Watanabe RG-1981

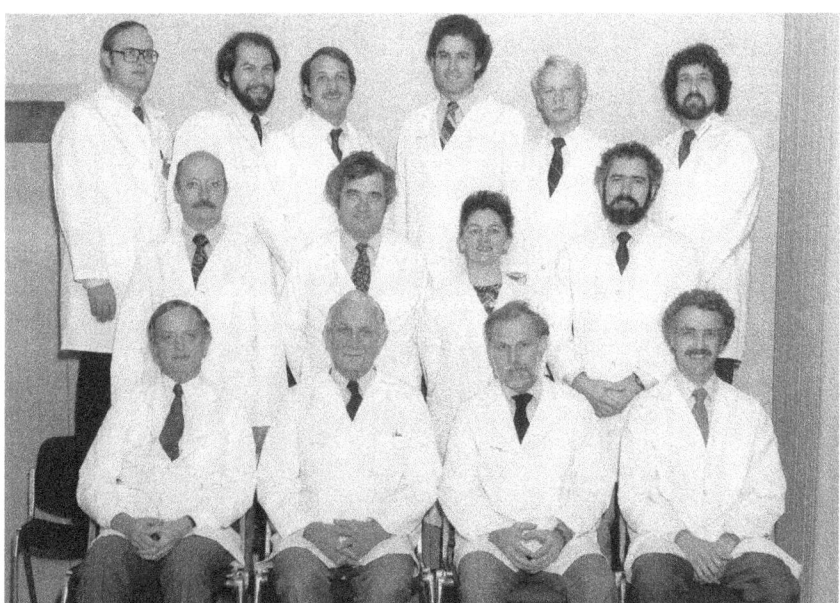

*Photo 1982:*

**FR:** Grabb, Dingman, Oneal, Markley (all TF)
**Second Row:** Newman TF; Cherry, Pasyk (both Lab); Izenberg TF
**Third Row:** Duus JR, Friedman 3&3, Derman JR, Marks RG-1982, Harder RG-1982, Gilman RG-1982

## 182  Group Images of Residents

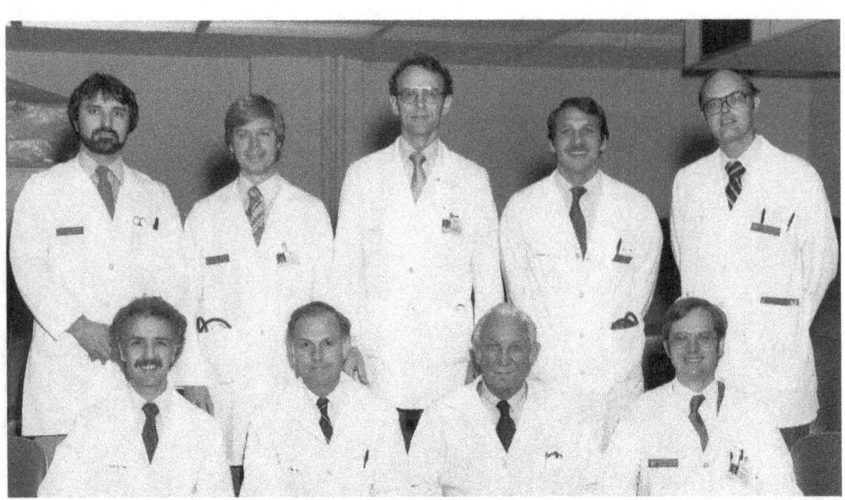

Photo 1983:

**FR:** Markley, Oneal, Dingman (now acting head), Stevenson (all TF)
**BR:** Rohrich 3&3, Zucker JR, Pollack JR, Derman RG-1983, Duus RG-1983

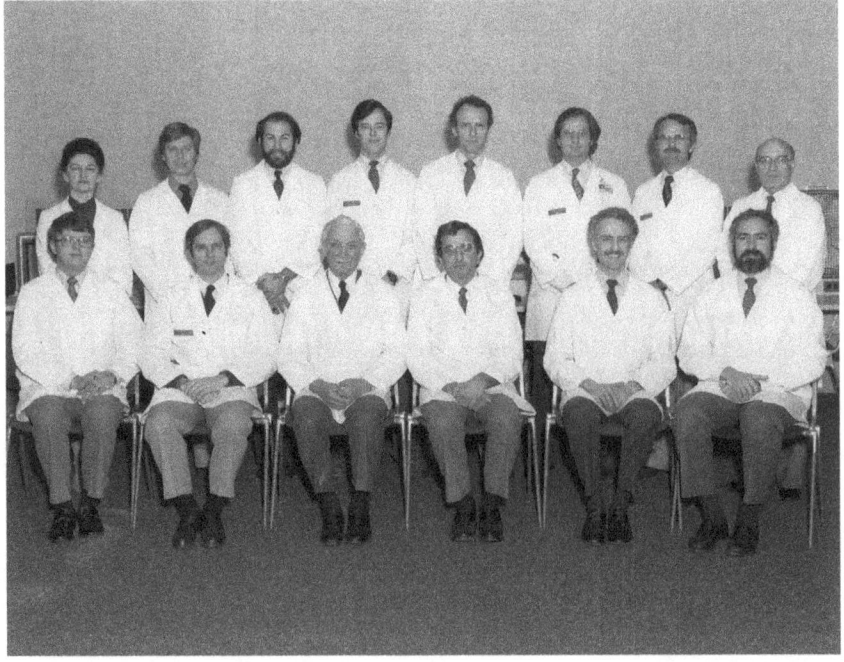

Photo 1984:

**FR:** Austad, Stevenson, Dingman, Argenta, Markley, Izenberg (all TF)
**BR:** Pasyk Lab, Zucker RG-1984, Friedman RG-1984, VanderKolk 3&3, Pollack RG-1984, Anderson JR, NI

# Leaders in Plastic Surgery 183

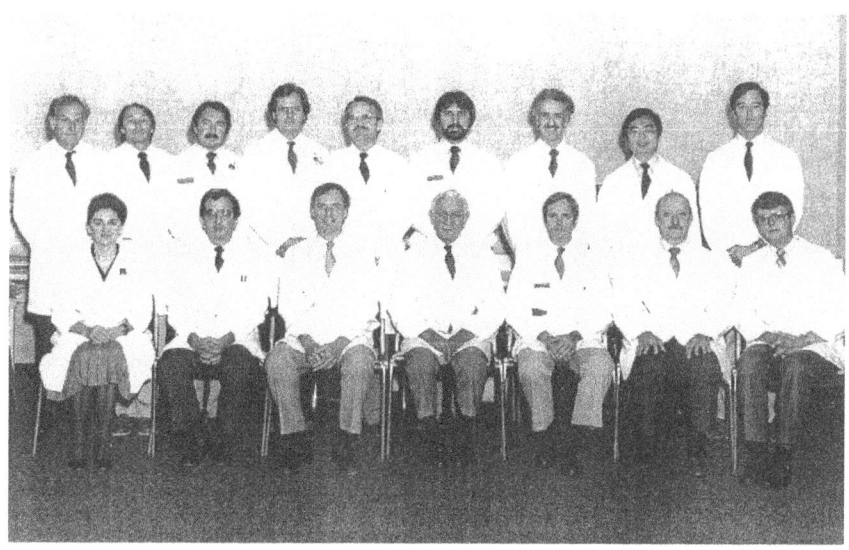

*Photo 1985:*

**FR:** Pasyk Lab; Argenta, Steve Mathes (now section head), Dingman, Stevenson, Newman, Austad (all TF)
**BR:** Oneal TF, Thornton JR, Adson JR, Hamm RG-1985, Anderson RG-1985, Rohrich RG-1985, Markley (TF), Fang, K., 3&3, VanderKolk JR

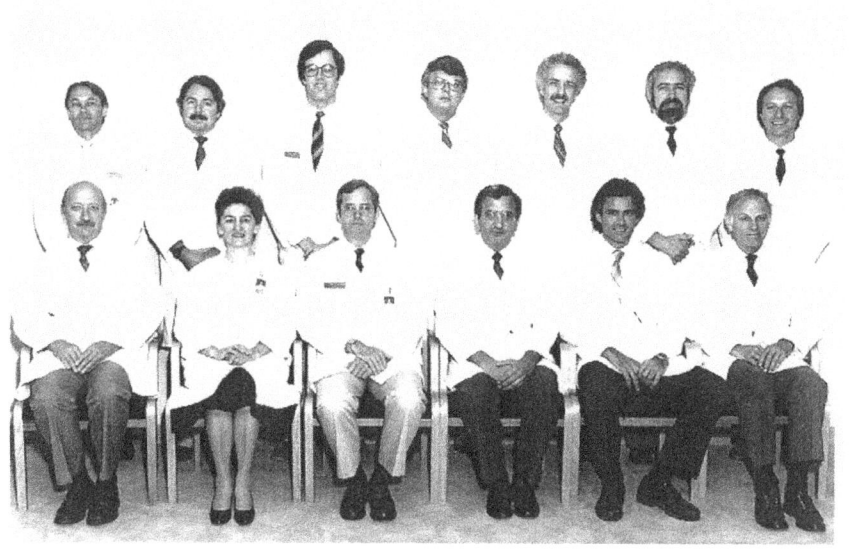

*Photo 1986:*

**FR:** Newman TF; Pasyk Lab; Stevenson, Argenta (now acting section head), Marks, Oneal (all TF)
**BR:** Thornton RG-1986; Adson RG-1986; VanderKolk RG-1986; Austad, Markley, Izenberg (all TF); Iacobucci JR

# References

### Chapter One

1 Reed O. Dingman, "A History of Plastic Surgery in the State of Michigan, the Early Years: 1918–1964" (presented before the Summer Meeting of the Michigan Academy of Plastic Surgeons, July 13–15, 1980).
2 Dingman, "A History of Plastic Surgery."
3 John Kemper, "The Responsibility of the Surgeon in Treating Palatal and Related Defects," Deep Blue, a division of the University of Michigan Library, http://deepblue.lib.umich.edu/bitstream/handle/2027.42/32568/0000694.pdf?sequence=1.
4 Dingman, "A History of Plastic Surgery."
5 David Dingman, personal communication, 2015.
6 Dingman, "A History of Plastic Surgery."

### Chapter Two

1 John Burke Tipton and Reed O. Dingman, "Some Aspects of Wound Healing in the Germfree Animal," *Plastic and Reconstructive Surgery* 38 (1966): 499.
2 Reed O. Dingman, Eulogy for William C. Grabb 1982.
3 Sir Harold Gillies and D. Ralph Millard, *Principles and Art of Plastic Surgery* (Boston: Little, Brown, 1957).

### Chapter Three

1 Lauralee Lutz, personal communication, 2010.
2 Ron Wexler, personal communication, 2015.
3 Plastic Surgery Plastic Surgery Section (PSS) Annual Reports, 1970–71; 1972–73.
4 Wexler, pers. comm.
5 John Markley, personal communication, 2010.
6 Ted Dodenhoff, personal communication, 2015.

### Chapter Four

1 Reed O. Dingman, PSS Annual Report 1973–74.
2 Reed O. Dingman, PSS Annual Report 1974–75.
3 Reed O. Dingman, "Trends in Medical Education in Relation to Plastic Surgery Residency Training," *Plastic and Reconstructive Surgery* 42 (1968): 292.
4 Cozette Grabb, (Mrs. William C. Grabb), personal communication, 2014.

5 William C. Grabb and James W. Smith, eds., *Plastic Surgery* (Boston: Little, Brown, 1968, 1973).
6 William C. Grabb, Sheldon Rosenstein, and Kenneth Bzoch, eds., *Cleft Lip and Palate* (Boston: Little, Brown, 1971).
7 Larry Berkowitz, personal communication, 2010.
8 Robert M. Oneal, Reed O. Dingman, and William C. Grabb, "Teaching of Plastic Surgical Techniques to Medical Students," *Plastic and Reconstructive Surgery* 40 (1967): 494.
9 Reed O. Dingman, PSS Annual Report, 1971–2.
10 William C. Grabb and Melvil Bert Myers, eds., *Skin Flaps* (Boston: Little, Brown, 1975).
11 Irving Feller and William C. Grabb, eds., *Reconstruction and Rehabilitation of Burns* (Ann Arbor: National Institute of Burn Medicine, 1979).
12 Louis Mes, personal communication, 2015.
13 Paul Izenberg, personal communication, 2014.
14 Robert Gilman, personal communication, 2015.
15 Lauralee Lutz, personal communication, 2014.
16 Gilman, pers. comm.
17 Feller and Grabb, eds., *Reconstruction and Rehabilitation of Burns*.
18 Lutz, pers. comm.
19 Gilman, pers. comm.
20 Malcolm Marks, personal communication, 2015.
21 Reed O. Dingman, Eulogy for William C. Grabb, 1982.
22 Lutz, pers. comm.
23 Marks, pers. comm.

## Chapter Five

1 Ted Dodenhoff, personal communication, 2015.
2 Issac Peled, personal communication, 2015.
3 Ernie Manders, personal communication, 2015.
4 Ross H. Musgrave, "A Variation on the Correction of the Congenital Lop Ear," *Plastic and Reconstructive Surgery* 37 (1966): 394.
5 Robert Wilensky, personal communication, 2010.
6 Dodenhoff, pers. comm.
7 Malcolm Marks, personal communication, 2015.
8 Grant R. Fairbanks, personal communication, 2010.
9 Don Davis, personal communication, 2010.
10 Robert D. Larsen and Robert M. Oneal, "The Use of Osteoperiosteal Flaps in Amputations in the Hand: Preliminary Report," *Plastic and Reconstructive Surgery* 38 (1966): 529.
11 Paul Izenberg, personal communication, 2015.
12 Ibid.
13 Louis Mes, personal communication, 2015.
14 Carl Berner, personal communication, 2015.
15 Manders, pers. comm.
16 Fairbanks, pers. comm.
17 Berner, pers. comm.

## Chapter Six

1 William C. Grabb, "The Experimental Method—An Editorial," *Plastic and Reconstructive Surgery* 49 (1972): 563.

2  John M. Markley, personal communication, 2014.
3  Paul Izenberg, personal communication, 2016.
4  Hassan Badran, personal communication, 2014.
5  Eric Austad, personal communication, 2015.
6  Neil F. Jones and Menachem Ron Wexler, "Delineation of the Pressure Sore Bursa Using Methylene Blue and Hydrogen Peroxide," *Plastic and Reconstructive Surgery* 68 (1981): 798.
7  Menachem Ron Wexler and Richard Faller, "Flap and Wound Size Tracing on Polyethylene Sheet," *Plastic and Reconstructive Surgery* 68 (1981): 103.
8  Menachem Ron Wexler, "An Arbor Flap: The Tree-Pattern Flap, or How Narrow May the Base of a Skin Flap Be? An Experimental Study," *Plastic and Reconstructive Surgery* 68 (1981): 185.
9  Menachem Ron Wexler, "Territorial Flooding, or Perfusion Takeover—An Experimental Study in Abdominal Flaps in the Pig," *Annals of Plastic Surgery* 8 (1982): 193.
10 Ron Wexler, personal communication, 2015.
11 Jim Norris, personal communication, 2014.
12 Lauralee Lutz, personal communication, 2015.
13 William C. Grabb, Spencer L. Bement, George H. Koepke, and Robert A. Green, "Comparison of Methods of Peripheral Nerve Suturing in Monkeys," *Plastic and Reconstructive Surgery* 46 (1970): 31.
14 C. Dennis Bucko, Robert L. Joynt, and William C. Grabb, "Peripheral Nerve Regeneration in Primates during D-Penicillamine-Induced Lathyrism," *Plastic and Reconstructive Surgery* 67 (1981): 23.
15 Dennis Bucko, personal communication, 2015.
16 Lutz, pers. comm.

## Chapter Seven

1  Reed O. Dingman, "Surgical Correction of Developmental Deformities of the Mandible," *Plastic and Reconstructive Surgery* 2 (1948): 124.
2  Reed O. Dingman, O. Lee Ricker, and Vivian Iob, "Blood Loss in Infant Cleft Lip and Cleft Palate Surgery," *Plastic and Reconstructive Surgery* 4 (1949): 333.
3  Reed O. Dingman, "Use of Iliac Bone in the Repair of Facial and Cranial Defects," *Plastic and Reconstructive Surgery* 6 (1950): 179.
4  Reed O. Dingman and Robert L. Harding, "Treatment of Malunion Fractures of Facial Bones," *Plastic and Reconstructive Surgery* 7 (1951): 505.
5  Reed O. Dingman, "Some Applications of the Z-Plasty Procedure," *Plastic and Reconstructive Surgery* 16 (1955): 246.
6  Reed O. Dingman, John D. Lynch, and Richard B. Asbury, "The Effectiveness of Sterilization of Canine Costal Cartilage by Cobalt 60 Irradiation and Its Fate when Used in Homografts," *Surgical Forum, Clinical Congress American College of Surgeons* 6 (1956): 581.
7  Reed O. Dingman, "Ostectomy of Mandible in the Habilitation of Cleft Lip and Palate Patients," *Plastic and Reconstructive Surgery* 25 (1960): 213.
8  Reed O. Dingman, "Correction of Nasal Deformities due to Defects of the Septum," *Plastic and Reconstructive Surgery* 18 (1956): 291.
9  Reed O. Dingman and William C. Grabb, "Lymphangioma of the Tongue," *Plastic and Reconstructive Surgery* 28(1961): 562.
10 Reed O. Dingman and William C. Grabb, "Costal Cartilage Homografts Preserved by Irradiation," *Plastic and Reconstructive Surgery* 28 (1961): 562.
11 Dingman, Lynch, and Asbury, "The Effectiveness of Sterilization of Canine Costal Cartilage by Cobalt 60 Irradiation."

12 Dingman and Grabb, "Costal Cartilage Homografts."
13 Ron Wexler, personal communication, 2015.
14 Paul Izenberg, personal communication, 2015.
15 Ibid.
16 Reed O. Dingman, "Necrobiosis Lipoidica Diabeticorum," *AMA Archives of Dermatology Syphalology* 63 (1951): 764.
17 Reed O. Dingman, Malunion of the Zygoma in the Transactions of the American Academy of Ophthalmology 1953: 889–896.
18 Donald F. Huelke, William C. Grabb, Reed O. Dingman, and Robert M. Oneal, "The New Automobile Windshield and Its Effectiveness in Reducing Facial Lacerations," *Plastic and Reconstructive Surgery* 41 (1968): 179.
19 Reed O. Dingman, "A New Instrument for Grasping Cartilage and Bone Grafts," *Plastic and Reconstructive Surgery* 14 (1954): 165.
20 Reed O. Dingman, Paul Natvig, and James M. Winkler, "A New Dressing Cart for Plastic Surgery," *Plastic and Reconstructive Surgery* 19 (1957): 72.
21 Reed O. Dingman and William C. Grabb, "A New Mouth Gag," *Plastic and Reconstructive Surgery* 29 (1962): 208.
22 Reed O. Dingman and William C. Grabb, "Reconstruction of Both Mandibular Condyles with Metatarsal Bone Grafts," *Plastic and Reconstructive Surgery* 34 (1964): 441.
23 Reed O. Dingman and William C. Grabb, "Surgical Anatomy of the Mandibular Ramus of the Facial Nerve Based upon the Dissection of 100 Facial Halves," *Plastic and Reconstructive Surgery* 29 (1962): 266.
24 William C. Grabb, "The First and Second Branchial Arch Syndrome," *Plastic and Reconstructive Surgery* 36 (1965): 485.
25 William C. Grabb, Reed O. Dingman, and Robert M. Oneal, "Flexor Tendon Grafts in the Hand," *Michigan Medicine* 66 (1967): 572.
26 John M. Markley, personal communication, 2014.
27 Ibid.
28 John M. Markley, "The Preservation of Close Two-Point Discrimination in Interdigital Transfer of Neurovascular Island Transfers," *Plastic and Reconstructive Surgery* 59 (1977): 812.
29 William C. Grabb, Reed O. Dingman, John Jesselson, J. R. Seaton, and Robert M. Oneal, "Statistical Evaluation of the Treatment of Basal Cell and Squamous Cell Carcinoma," *University of Michigan Medical Center Journal* 35 (1969): 204.
30 William C. Grabb, Malcolm S. MacCollum, and Nick G. Tan, "Results from Tattooing Port-Wine Hemangiomas," *Plastic and Reconstructive Surgery* 59 (1977): 667.
31 Malcolm W. Marks, Louis C. Argenta, and Reed O. Dingman, "Traumatic Arteriovenous Malformation of the External Carotid Arterial System," *Head and Neck Surgery* 6 (l984): 1054.
32 Krystyna A. Pasyk, Reed O. Dingman, Louis C. Argenta, and Gary S. Sandall, "The Management of Hemangiomas of the Head and Neck," *Head and Neck Surgery* 6 (1984): 851.
33 William C. Grabb and Robert M. Oneal, "The Effect of Molecular Eight Dextran on the Survival of Experimental Skin Flaps," *Plastic and Reconstructive Surgery* 37 (1966): 406.
34 Robert M. Oneal, Robert E. Knode, William C. Grabb, and Reed O. Dingman, "The Effect of Low Molecular Weight Dextran on the Survival of Skin Flaps Vascularized Either by a Single Artery and Vein or by a Subdermal Plexus," *Plastic and Reconstructive Surgery* 40 (1967): 595.

35 Robert J. Wilensky and William C. Grabb, "Soft Tissue Coverage of the Lower Extremities," *Michigan Medicine* 74 (1975): 592.
36 William C. Grabb and Melvil Bert Myers, eds., *Skin Flaps* (Boston: Little, Brown, 1975).
37 Ibid.
38 Frank McDowell, from the Foreword in Grabb and Myers, *Skin Flaps*.
39 Grabb and Myers, *Skin Flaps*.
40 S. H. Milton, "Fallacy of the Length-Width Ratio," *British Journal of Surgery* 57 (1970): 502.
41 Grabb and Myers, *Skin Flaps*.
42 Berish Strauch, Luis O. Vasconez, Elizabeth Hall-Findlay, and William C. Grabb, *Grabb's Encyclopedia of Flaps* (Boston: Little, Brown, 1990).
43 Grabb and Myers, *Skin Flaps*.
44 Sigurdur E. Thorvaldsson and William C. Grabb, "The Intravenous Fluorescein Test as a Measure of Skin Flap Viability," *Plastic and Reconstructive Surgery* 53 (1974): 576.
45 Paul Izenberg, personal communication later in 2016.
46 Leonard T. Furlow, "Editorial," *Annals of Plastic Surgery* 73 (2014): 1.
47 Ibid.
48 John McCraw and Phillip G. Arnold, *Atlas of Muscle and Myocutaneous Flaps* (Hampton Press, 1986).
49 Stephen J. Mathes, Luis O. Vasconez, and Maurice J. Jurkiewicz, "Extensions and Further Applications of Muscle Flap Transposition," *Plastic and Reconstructive Surgery* 60 (1977): 6.
50 John B. McCraw, David G. Dibble, and James H. Carraway, "Clinical Definition of Independent Myocutaneous Vascular Territories," *Plastic and Reconstructive Surgery* 60 (1977): 341.
51 Stephen J. Mathes and Foad Nahai, *Clinical Atlas of Muscle and Myocutaneous Flaps* (St. Louis: Mosby, 1979).
52 Paul Izenberg, personal communication, 2016.
53 Ibid.
54 Paul Izenberg, personal communication later in 2016.
55 Plastic Surgery PSS Annual Reports, 1970–71; 1972–73.
56 Jim Norris, personal communication, 2014.
57 Reed O. Dingman, PSS Annual Report 1973–4.
58 Markley, pers. comm.
59 Ernie Manders, personal communication, 2015.
60 Robert Gilman, personal communication, 2016.
61 Paul Izenberg, personal communication later in 2016.
62 Ibid.
63 Eric Austad, personal communication, 2015.
64 Robert M. Oneal, Rod J. Rohrich, and Paul H. Izenberg, "Skin Expansion as an Adjunct to Reconstruction of the External Ear," *British Journal of Plastic Surgery* 37 (1984): 517.
65 J. O. Strombeck, "Mammoplasty: Report of a New Technique Based on the Two-Pedicle Procedure," *British Journal of Plastic Surgery* 13 (1960): 79.
66 Paul K. McKissock, "Reduction Mammoplasty with a Vertical Dermal Flap," *Plastic and Reconstructive Surgery* 49 (1971): 245.
67 E. H. Courtiss and R. M. Goldwyn, "A Reduction Mammoplasty by the Inferior Pedicle Technique," *Plastic and Reconstructive Surgery* 59 (1977): 500.
68 E. H. Courtiss and R. M. Goldwyn, "Update on Inferior Pedicle Reduction," *Plastic and Reconstructive Surgery* 66 (1980): 646.

69 Daniel Marchac and G. de Olarte, "Reduction Mammaplasty and Correction of Ptosis with a Short Inframammary Scar," *Plastic and Reconstructive Surgery* 69 (1982): 45.
70 T. D. Cronin and F. T. Gerow, "Augmentation Mammoplasty: A New 'Natural Feel' Prosthesis" (Transactions of the Third International Congress of Plastic Surgery, Excerpta Medica, Amsterdam, 1963).
71 Robert M. Oneal, letter to the editor, "High-Pressure Injection of Silicone into Axilla—A Complication of Closed Compression Capsulotomy of the Breast," *Plastic and Reconstructive Surgery* 64 (1979): 700.
72 Robert M. Oneal and Louis C. Argenta, "Late Side Effects Related to Inflatable Breast Prostheses Containing Soluble Steroids," *Plastic and Reconstructive Surgery* 66 (1982): 641.
73 Robert M. Oneal, "Reply in Correspondence Section: Side Effects of Solumedrol Placed in Breast Prostheses Containing Soluble Steroids," *Plastic and Reconstructive Surgery* 71 (1983): 283.
74 K. L. Pickrell, C. L. Puckett, and K. S. Given, "Subpectoral Augmentation Mammoplasty," *Plastic and Reconstructive Surgery* 62 (1978): 706.
75 Tom Hudak, personal communication, 2015.
76 Joseph Agris, Reed O. Dingman, and Robert J. Wilensky, "A Dissector for Transaxillary Approach in Augmentation," *Plastic and Reconstructive Surgery* 57 (1976): 10.
77 John R. Jarrett, Ralph G. Cutler, and Donald F. Teal, "Subcutaneous Mastectomy in Small, Large or Ptotic Breasts with Immediate Submuscular Placement of Implants," *Plastic and Reconstructive Surgery* 62 (1978): 702.
78 Paul Izenberg, personal communication later in 2016.
79 Ibid.
80 Ibid.
81 Ibid.
82 C. R. Hartrampf, Michael Sheflan, and Paul W. Black, "Breast Reconstruction with a Transverse Abdominal Island Flap," *Plastic and Reconstructive Surgery* 69 (1982): 216.
83 Roger Friedman, Louis Argenta, and Richard Anderson, "Case Report: Deep Inferior Epigastric Free Flap for Breast Reconstruction Post Mastectomy," *Plastic and Reconstructive Surgery* 76 (1985): 455.
84 Menachem Ron Wexler and Robert M. Oneal, "Areolar Sharing to Reconstruct the Absent Nipple," *Plastic and Reconstructive Surgery* 51 (1972): 176.
85 William C. Grabb, Sheldon Rosenstein, and Kenneth Bzoch, eds., *Cleft Lip and Palate* (Boston: Little, Brown, 1971).
86 John Kemper, "The Responsibility of the Surgeon in Treating Palatal and Related Defects," http://deepblue.lib.umich.edu/bitstream/handle/2027.42/32568/0000694.pdf?sequence=1.
87 D. Ralph Millard, "Refinements in Rotation-Advancement Cleft Lip Technique," *Plastic and Reconstructive Surgery* 33 (1964): 26.
88 Ernie Kaplan, personal communication, 1974.
89 Robert Pool, personal communication, 1979.
90 Robert Pool, "The Configuration of the Unilateral Cleft Lip with Reference to Rotation Advancement Surgery," *Plastic and Reconstructive Surgery* 37 (1966): 558.
91 D. Ralph Millard Jr., "Closure of Bilateral Cleft Lip and Elongation of Columella by Two Operations in Infancy," *Plastic and Reconstructive Surgery* 47 (1971): 324.
92 Robert M. Oneal, Donald M. Greer, and Gary L. Nobel, "Secondary Correction of Bilateral Cleft Deformities with Millard's Midline Muscular Closure," *Plastic and Reconstructive Surgery* 54 (1974): 45.

93 D. Ralph Millard Jr., *Bilateral and Rare Deformities*, Cleft Craft, vol II (Boston: Little, Brown, 1977).
94 Reed O. Dingman and William C. Grabb, "Complexities of Bilateral Cleft Lip and Palate," *Plastic and Reconstructive Surgery* 47 (1971): 239.
95 Dingman and Grabb, "A New Mouth Gag."
96 Richard Sarns, personal communication, 2016.
97 Leonard T. Furlow, "Cleft Palate Repair by Double Opposing Z-Plasty," *Plastic and Reconstructive Surgery* 78 (1986): 724 Originally described in D. Ralph Millard, *Alveolar and Palatal Deformities*, Cleft Craft, vol III (Boston: Little, Brown, 1980), pp. 519–20.
98 Plastic Surgery PSS Annual Reports, 1970–71; 1972–73.
99 D. Ralph Millard, *Alveolar and Palatal Deformities*, Cleft Craft, vol III (Boston: Little, Brown, 1980), p. 1014.
100 R. A. Latham, R. P. Kusy, and N. G. Georgiade, "An Externally Activated Appliance for Cleft Palate Infants," *Cleft Palate-Craniofacial Journal* 13 (1976): 253.
101 Harold McComb, "Treatment of the Unilateral Cleft Lip Nose," *Plastic and Reconstructive Surgery* 55 (1975): 596.
102 Harold McComb, "Primary Correction of the Unilateral Cleft Lip Nose. A 15 Year Review," *Plastic and Reconstructive Surgery* 75 (1985): 791.
103 Miguel Orticochea, "Construction of a Dynamic Muscle Sphincter in Cleft Palates," *Plastic and Reconstructive Surgery* 41 (1968): 323.
104 Ian T. Jackson and John S. Silverton, "The Sphincter Pharyngoplasty as a Secondary Procedure in Cleft Palates," *Plastic and Reconstructive Surgery* 59 (1977): 518.
105 Robert M. Oneal, Paul H. Izenberg, Rod J. Rohrich, and Craig A. VanderKolk, "The Use of Naso-Endoscopy Diagnosis and Management of Velo-Pharyngeal Insufficiency," in *Surgical Endoscopy*, ed. T. Dent, W. E. Strodel, and J. G. Turcotte (Chicago: Year book Publishers, 1985).
106 Ray Fonseca, personal communication.
107 Carl Berner, personal communication, 2015.
108 Reed O. Dingman, personal communication, 1971.
109 Jack Sheen, "Secondary Rhinoplasty," *Plastic and Reconstructive Surgery* 56 (1975): 135.
110 Reed O. Dingman and Paul Natvig, "The Infra-cartilaginous Incision for Rhinoplasty," *Plastic and Reconstructive Surgery* 69 (1982): 134.
111 Sten J. Stenstrom, "A 'Natural' Technique for Correction of Congenitally Prominent Ears," *Plastic and Reconstructive Surgery* 32 (1963): 135.
112 J. C. Mustarde, "Correction of Prominent Ears Using Simple Mattress Sutures," *British Journal of Plastic Surgery* 16 (1963): 170.
113 Reed O. Dingman and Isaac Peled, "Corrective Cosmetic Otoplasty: A Simple and Accurate Technique," *Annals of Plastic Surgery* 3 (1979): 250.
114 David W. Furnas, "Correction of Prominent Ears by Concha-Mastoid Sutures," *Plastic and Reconstructive Surgery* 42 (1968): 189.
115 Tord Skoog, *Plastic Surgery* (Stockholm: Almqvist and Wiksell, 1974).
116 V. Mitz and M. Peyronie, "The Superficial Musculo-Aponeurotic System (SMAS) in the Parotid and Cheek Area," *Plastic and Reconstructive Surgery* 58 (1976): 80.
117 Daniel C. Baker, personal communication at ASPRS meeting.
118 Daniel C. Baker and John Conley, "Avoiding Facial Nerve Injuries in Rhytidectomy," *Plastic and Reconstructive Surgery* 64 (1979): 781.
119 Peter McKinney and David J. Katrana, "Prevention of Injury to the Great Auricular Nerve in Rhytidectomy," *Plastic and Reconstructive Surgery* 66 (1980): 675.

120 Menachem Ron Wexler, "Notes on Male Rhytidectomy," *Chirurgia Plastica* 4 (1977): 51.
121 Marcia K. Goin, R. W. Burgoyne, and John M. Goin, "A Prospective Study of 50 Female Face-Lift Patients," *Plastic and Reconstructive Surgery* 65 (1980): 436.
122 Thomas D. Rees, David M. Liverett, and Cary L. Guy, "The Effect of Cigarette Smoking on Skin-Flap Survival in Face-Lift Patients," *Plastic and Reconstructive Surgery* 73 (1984): 911.
123 Reed O. Dingman, I. Peled, and Paul H. Izenberg, "Forehead and Browlift and Their Relationship to Blepharoplasty," *Annals of Plastic Surgery* 2 (1979): 32.
124 S. Castanares, "Blepharoplasty for Herniated Intraorbital Fat. Anatomic Basis for a New Approach," *Plastic and Reconstructive Surgery* 8 (1951): 46.
125 John Clarke Mustarde, *Repair and Reconstruction in the Orbital Region* (Baltimore: Williams and Wilkins, 1966).
126 Ulrich K. Kessering and Rodolphe Meyer, "A Suction Curette for Removal of Excessive Local Deposits of Subcutaneous Fat," *Plastic and Reconstructive Surgery* 62 (1978): 305.
127 Yves-Gerard Illouz, "Body Contouring by Lipolysis: A 5 Year Experience with over 3000 Cases," *Plastic and Reconstructive Surgery* 72 (1983): 591.
128 Reed O. Dingman and Paul Natvig, *Surgery of Facial Fractures* (Philadelphia: W.B. Saunders, 1964).
129 C. Gardner Child, quote from preface of *Surgery of Facial Fractures*.
130 G. Kasten Tallmadge, quote from epilogue of *Surgery of Facial Fractures*.
131 Reed O. Dingman, William C. Grabb, and Robert M. Oneal, "Management of Injuries of the Naso-Orbital Complex," *Archives of Surgery* 98 (1969): 566.
132 Reed O. Dingman and Paul H. Izenberg, "Complications of Facial Trauma," in *Complications of Head and Neck Surgery*, ed. John Conley (Philadelphia: W.B. Sanders, 1979), 353.
133 Reed O. Dingman, William C. Grabb, Robert M. Oneal, and Robert Ponitz, "Sternocleidomastoid Muscle Transplant to the Master Area," *Plastic and Reconstructive Surgery* 43 (1969): 5.
134 Hudak, pers. comm.
135 Reed O. Dingman and E. Constant, "A Fifteen Experience with Temporomandibular Diseases," *Plastic and Reconstructive Surgery* 44 (1969): 119
136 Reed O. Dingman, David L. Dingman, and Richard A. Lawrence, "Surgical Correction of Lesions of the Temporomandibular Joint," *Plastic and Reconstructive Surgery* 55 (1975): 335.
137 David Dingman, personal communication, 2015.
138 Leonard Glass, personal communication, 2015.
139 Bruce Novark, personal communication, 2015.
140 Menachem Ron Wexler and Reed O. Dingman, "Construction of the Lower Lip," *Chirugia Plastica* 3 (1975): 23.
141 Grant R. Fairbanks, personal communication, 2010.
142 Reed O. Dingman and Grant R. Fairbanks, "Restoration of the Oral Commissure," *Plastic and Reconstructive Surgery* 49 (1972): 411.
143 P. Tessier, "Total Osteotomies of the Face: Crouzon Syndrome," *Annales de Chirurgie Plastique Esthétique* 12 (1967): 272.
144 Haskell Newman, personal communication, 2015.
145 Glass, pers. comm.
146 Newman, pers. comm.
147 Hudak, pers. comm.

148 Wexler, pers. comm.
149 Newman, pers. comm.

## Chapter Eight

1 Grant R. Fairbanks, personal communication, 2010.
2 Reed O. Dingman, "A History of Plastic Surgery in the State of Michigan, the Early Years: 1918–1964" (presented before the Summer Meeting of the Michigan Academy of Plastic Surgeons, July 13–15, 1980).

## Chapter Nine

1 Ernie Manders, personal communication, 2015.
2 Paul Izenberg, personal communication, 2015.
3 Manders, pers. comm.
4 Bruce Novark, personal communication, 2010.
5 Bruce Novark, personal communication, 2015.
6 Larry Berkowitz, personal communication, 2010.
7 Hudak, Ibid.
8 Richard Anderson, personal communication, 2015.
9 Ron Wexler, personal communication, 2015.
10 Issac Peled, personal communication, 2015.
11 Leonard Glass, personal communication, 2015.
12 Anderson, pers. comm.
13 Izenberg, pers. comm.
14 Grant R. Fairbanks, personal communication, 2010.
15 James Stilwell, personal communication, 2015.
16 Jim Norris, personal communication, 2014.
17 Ibid.
18 Manders, pers. comm.
19 Lauralee Lutz, personal communication, 2010.
20 Robert Wilensky, personal communication, 2010.
21 Ted Dodenhoff, personal communication, 2015.
22 Wexler, pers. comm.
23 Norris, pers. comm.
24 Lutz, pers. comm., 2010.
25 Mes, pers. comm., 2010.
26 Wilensky, pers. comm.
27 Fairbanks, pers. comm.
28 Leonard Glass, personal communication, 2010.
29 Fairbanks, pers. comm.
30 Peled, pers. comm.
31 Don Greer, personal communication, 2010.
32 Novark, pers. comm., 2015.
33 Manders, pers. comm.
34 Lauralee Lutz, personal communication, 2014.
35 Ibid.
36 D. Ralph Millard, *Alveolar and Palatal Deformities*, Cleft Craft, vol III (Boston: Little, Brown, 1980), p. 1013.
37 Malcolm Marks, quoted remarks at ROD Society Meeting, Ann Arbor, MI, 2007.
38 Ibid.
39 Lauralee Lutz, personal communication, 2015.

40 Reed O. Dingman, William C. Grabb, Robert M. Oneal, and Robert Ponitz, "Sternocleidomastoid Muscle Transplant to the Master Area," *Plastic and Reconstructive Surgery* 43:5, 44:119, 1969.
41 Peled, pers. comm.
42 Fairbanks, pers. comm.
43 Lauralee Lutz, personal communication, from her own notes given to me in 2010.
44 Novark, pers. comm., 2015.
45 Peled, pers. comm.
46 Manders, pers. comm.
47 Lauralee Lutz, "Shakespeare on Plastic Surgery," *Plastic and Reconstructive Surgery* 74 (1984): 841.
48 Don Ditmars, personal communication, 2016.
49 Greer, pers. comm.
50 Novark, pers. comm., 2015.
51 Norris, pers. comm.
52 Fairbanks, pers. comm.
53 Harvey Weiss, A Remarkable Mentor, Letter in Medicine at Michigan, Spring 2006, p. 4.

## Epilogue

1 Malcolm Marks, personal communication, 2015.
2 Ibid.
3 Allison Wilson, "Humanizing Prosthetics," *Medicine at Michigan*, Summer 2015, 14.
4 David Brown, Gregory Borschel, Benjamin Levi, and Shoshana Woo, *Michigan Manual of Plastic Surgery* (Philadelphia: Wolters Kluwer, 2016).

## Appendix

1 Elbert Hubbard, *A Message to Garcia* (New York: Peter Pauper Press, 1982).
2 Sigurdur E. Thorvaldsson, "Icelandic Journey," *Annals of Plastic Surgery* 48 (2002): 556.

# About the Authors

**Robert M. Oneal, MD** was born in Evanston, Illinois, and grew up in nearby Wilmette until age eighteen. After graduation from New Trier High School, he attended Dartmouth College in Hanover, New Hampshire, where he also completed his first two years in medical school, and then obtained his MD degree at Harvard Medical School in Boston. He completed a general surgery residency and then a plastic surgery residency in Ann Arbor, Michigan. He has been an active faculty member in the Section of Plastic Surgery at the University of Michigan since 1966, rising to the position of clinical professor and was in private practice at Saint Joseph Mercy Hospital (SJMH) for forty years. Since retirement in 2006, he has continued teaching plastic surgery residents, living in Ann Arbor with his wife and author, Zibby Oneal.

**Lauralee Lutz** was born near State College, Pennsylvania, and grew in Connecticut, earning her BA in English and botany from Connecticut College in New London. Her early work includes being the horticultural advisor to a major Connecticut nursery where she also developed a newspaper column and radio program on gardening. Later she moved to Michigan where she worked in various hospital laboratories until joining the Section of Plastic Surgery as secretary and administrator. Her organizational skills and personality fit well in this niche for more than twenty years.

# Index

**A**
Abbe flap, 98
Agris, J., 71, 93
alprazolam (Xanax), 43
alveolar bone grafts, 103–104
*AMA Archives of Dermatology and Syphilology*, 68
amblyopia, 77
ambulatory surgical facility (ASF), 44
American Board of Plastic Surgery, 12
American Society of Plastic and Reconstructive Surgery (ASPRS), 26, 46
Anderson, Jack, 106
Anderson, Richard, 22, 95, 128, 129
  Ann Arbor plastic surgery experience, 128
Ann Arbor Veterans Administration Hospital (VA)
  Henry Ford Hospital (HFH) and rotations of its residents, 152
  Plastic Surgery Residency Training, 150–152
  research laboratory, 53
  resident rotations at, 48–49
*Archives of Otolaryngology*, 66
Argenta, Louis, 32, 38, 76, 85, 92, 95, 146, 148
  breast augmentation and, 92
  clinical skin expansion and, 88
Arnold, P. G., 80
  *Atlas of Muscle and Myocutaneous Flaps*, 80
Asbury, Richard B., 66
Austad, Eric, 33, 55, 62, 88
  clinical skin expansion and, 87–88
  face-lifting and, 109
  skin flaps and, 63
  tissue expansion, development of, 57–58

**B**
Badran, Hassan, 57
Baker, Daniel, 108
Balloon Federation of America, 139
Bartlett, Robert, 84
basal cell lesions, 75
Bement, Spencer L., 64
Bennett, Jim, 71
Berkowitz, Larry, 27, 128
  Ann Arbor plastic surgery experience, 127–128
  myocutaneous (musculocutaneous) flaps and, 80–81
Berner, Carl, 22, 48, 104
Bethea, Hardy, 124
bilateral cleft lip (BCL), 98–99
Billman, Howard, 4
Black, Paul W., 95
blepharoplasty, 43, 109–110
Blocksma, Ralph, 124
Bloomer, Harlan, 70, 101
Bloom, Herbert, 117
Braley, Silas, 58
branchial arch syndrome, first and second, 71
breast augmentation, 90–93
breast reconstruction, 94–95
breast surgery
  breast augmentation, 90–93
  breast reconstruction, 94–95
  prophylactic mastectomy, 93–94
  reduction mammoplasty, 89–90
brow-lifting, 109–110
Buatti, Gene, 101
Bucko, Dennis, 30–31, 64, 65
Buncke, Harry, 21
Burgoyne, R. W., 109
Buxton, Robert, 21
Byrd, Steve, 106
Bzoch, Kenneth, 95

195

## C

Carlson, Bruce, 148
Carraway, James H., 80
Castanares, S., 110
Cederna, Paul, 147–148
Cerny, Joseph, 86
certified registered nurse anesthetists (CRNAs), 43
Chase, Robert, 19
cheilitis glandularis, 68
Cherry, George, 55, 61, 88
  skin flaps and, 62
Child, C. Gardner, 112
Child III, Charles Gardner, 12–13, 24
  facial fractures AND, 112
*Cleft Craft*, 98
cleft lip and palate, 95–104
  alveolar bone grafts, 103–104
  bilateral cleft lip, 98–99
  cleft palate, 99–101
  cleft palate clinics, 101
  nasoendoscopy, 103
  presurgical palatal orthopedics, 101–102
  UCL nose, 102–103
  unilateral cleft lip, 96–98, 152
*Cleft Lip and Palate: One Saturday Morning a Month*, 51–52
*Cleft Lip and Palate: Surgical, Dental, and Speech Aspects*, 26, 95
cleft palate, 99–101
  clinics, 101
Clifford, Robert, 124, 152
*Clinical Atlas of Muscle and Musculocutaneous Flaps, The*, 80
clinical microvascular surgery, 83–85
clinical skin expansion, 87–88
Coller, Frederick A., 5, 7
congenital capillary (strawberry) hemangioma, 76–77
congenital protruding ear deformity, 107
Conley, John, 108, 113
Constant, E., 71, 115
Converse, John M., 31
  craniofacial surgery and, 118
Courtiss, E. H., 89, 90
Cozy, Bill, 26
craniofacial surgery, 117–119
Cronin, T. D., 90
Curtis, Arthur "Whitey," 68
cutaneous vascular lesions, treatment of, 76–77
Cutler, Ralph G., 93

## D

Daniel, Rollin, 78
David, Dingman
  maxillofacial surgery and, 115–116
David Furnas, 107
Davis, Don, 46
Davis, Don G., 13, 46, 71
decubitus ulcers, treatment of, 81–83
deltopectoral flap, 85
Dempsey, Paul, 71
  face-lifting and, 109
de Olarte, G., 90
dermal tattooing, 76
Derman, *Plastic Surgery*, 85
diazepam (Valium), 43
Dibble, David G., 80
Dingman, David, 2, 4, 21–22, 115, 116
  eulogy for his father, 169
Dingman mouth gag, 99
Dingman, Reed O. (ROD), 1, 2–5, 7–9, 11–16, 18, 19–20, 24, 25, 26, 27, 28, 31, 33, 35–37, 39, 66, 67, 68, 69, 71, 72, 74, 76, 77, 82, 93, 99, 105, 107, 109, 111, 112, 113, 115, 117, 125, 142, 153
  *Archives of Surgery*, 113
  bilateral cleft lip and, 99
  blepharoplasty and, 109–110
  brow-lifting and, 109–110
  cleft palate and, 100
  clinical microvascular surgery and, 84
  congenital protruding ear deformity and, 107
  craniofacial surgery and, 118
  decubitus ulcers and, 82–83
  early work of, 66–71
  eulogy by Dingman, David L. for, 169
  face-lifting and, 108
  graduations, 135
  Lauralee's eulogy letter for, 168
  letter from Lutz, 163
  letter to Grabb, 158
  lip reconstruction and, 117
  maxillofacial surgery and, 114–116
  motto, quotations, and advice to residents, 166–167

Oneal's eulogy for, 171–173
outside activities of, 131–132
personal anecdotes/adages, 133
photography, 134–135
quotes from Osler, 164–165
resident rotations and, 40–43, 45, 48, 130
resident selection experience, 130–131
retirement as Section of Plastic Surgery head, 23–26
rhinoplasty and, 104, 105
at Saturday morning teaching rounds, 50
*Surgery of Facial Fractures*, 70, 112–113
TMJ reconstruction with metatarsal grafts, 69–70
Ditmars, Don, 143–144, 152
Dodenhoff, Ted, 21–22, 40, 43, 133
on Dingman, 133
Dow Corning Medical Products, 58–59
Duus, Erlan, 22, 106

E
Edgerton, Milton, 28
"Encyclopedia of Flaps, The," 35, 79
enhanced seatbelt reminder (ESBR), 112
Entin, Martin, 28
Ewing, Joseph, 4
"Experimental Method, The," 53–54
eyelid capillary hemangioma, 76

F
face-lifting, 107–109
facial disfigurement, prosthetic correction for, 16
facial fractures, 112–113
facial lacerations, 69
Facial Trauma, 52
Fairbanks, Grant, 22, 45, 48, 71, 117, 123, 130, 135, 136, 142, 144
  Ann Arbor rounds and conferences, 129–130
  on Dingman, 135, 136
  lip reconstruction and, 117
  on Oneal, 142
Faller, Richard, 63
  skin flaps and, 62–63
Faulkner, John, 56, 57, 148

Feller, I., 28, 29, 35, 40, 68
flap delay, 61
Fonseca, Ray, 104
forked flaps, 98, 99
Fralich, Bruce, 15
Friedman, Roger, 27, 95
F. Roland Sargent Research Laboratory, research activities at, 53–65
  nerve suturing techniques, in monkeys, 64–65
  skin flaps, 62–64
  tissue expansion, 57–62
Fryer, Minot, 3
Furlow, Leonard, 79, 100
Furnas, David W., 107

G
gender reassignment surgery, 86–87
Georgiade, N. G., 102
Gerow, F. T., 90
Gillies, Harold, 1, 9–10
  painting, 170
Gilman, Bob, 35, 71, 84–85
  rhinoplasty and, 106
Gilman, Robert, 22, 34–35, 85
Given, K. S., 92
Glass, Lenny, 22, 116, 129, 136
  Ann Arbor rounds and conferences, 129
  craniofacial surgery and, 118
  maxillofacial surgery and, 116
Goin, John M., 109
Goin, Marcia K., 109
Goldwyn, R. M., 89, 90
Gorney, Mark, 28–29
Grabb, Cozette, 26
Grabb, William C. (WCG, Bill), 7–8, 10, 13, 17, 18, 19, 25, 26, 27, 28, 29, 30, 35, 37, 53, 60, 64, 66, 67, 69, 71, 72, 74, 76, 77, 78, 79, 87, 88, 95, 99, 106, 113, 115, 137–142, 139, 153
  *Archives of Surgery*, 113
  bilateral cleft lip and, 99
  cleft palate and, 100–101
  clinical skin expansion and, 87
  death of, 34–38
  and Dingman, 36–37, 158
  early work of, 66–71
  "Encyclopedia of Flaps, The," 35, 79
  eulogy, by Oneal, 160

198  Index

"Experimental Method,
  The," 53–54
face-lifting and, 108
gender reassignment surgery and, 86
as head of Section of Plastic
  Surgery, 30
letter to Lennie, 159
as member of ASPRS Board of
  Directors, 26
memorial remarks from his
  residents, 161
as president of ASPRS Educational
  Foundation, 26
resident rotations and, 40, 43, 45, 47
skin flaps and, 62–64, 77–78, 79
"Ten Most Wanted" Lists, 156–157
as tenure of Section of Plastic
  Surgery head, 26–30
at Thursday morning
  conference, 50
TMJ reconstruction with
  metatarsal grafts, 69–70
at weekly Saturday morning
  research conference, 51
"Great Rift, The" (painting by
  Gillies), 170
Greenfield, Laser, 146
Green, Robert A., 64
Greer, D., 77, 98, 136, 148
  on Dingman, 136
  on Lauralee, 144
Gronvall, John A., 23
Gunter, Jack, 22
  rhinoplasty and, 105, 106
Guy, Cary L., 109

H
Hall-Findlay, Elizabeth, 79
Halsted mastectomy, 57
Hamm, Jeffrey, 27
Hand Conference, 52
hand joint replacement with silicone
  implants, 74
hand rotation, in Detroit, 45–46
hand surgery, 72–74
Hansen, Wilmer, 4
Harder, Glenn, 27
Harding, Robert L., 66
Harrell, Eugene, 46
Hartrampf, C. R., 95
Hayward, James, 12, 100
Henry Ford Hospital (HFH), and
  resident rotators, 152

Hertel, Richard, 86
Hodge, Gerald P., 15, 16, 70–71
Hodge, Jerry, 52
Hopkins, Johns, 30
Hubbard, Elbert, 36, 162
Hudak, T., 22, 92, 115, 118
  Ann Arbor plastic surgery
    experience, 128
Huelke, Donald, 69, 70
"Hunter silicone rod" technique, 72

I
Illouz, Yves-Gerard, 111
images of residents, 174–183
interphalangeal joint (IPJ) implants, 74
Iob, Vivian, 66
Isaac Peled, 107
Ivy, Robert H., 26
Izenberg, Paul, 18, 33, 46, 47, 48,
    57, 68, 71, 80, 81, 85, 86, 88,
    94, 103, 109, 113, 127,
    129, 141
  Ann Arbor plastic surgery
    experience, 127
  Ann Arbor rounds and
    conferences, 129
  breast reconstruction and, 94–95
  cartilage homografts and, 68
  clinical microvascular surgery
    and, 85
  clinical skin expansion and, 88
  decubitus ulcers and, 81
  face-fractures and, 113
  face-lifting and, 109
  myocutaneous (musculocutaneous)
    flaps and, 80–81
  rat hind limb arterial anastomosis
    patency model, 57
  resident rotations and, 43, 47
  rhinoplasty and, 106
  shotgun injuries to the face
    and, 85–86

J
Jackson, Ian T., 103
Jaffee, Bob, 86
Jarrett, John R., 93
Jesselson, John, 74
John Mustarde, 107, 111
  *Repair and Reconstruction in the
    Orbital Region*, 110
Joint Commission on Residency
  Training, 6

Jones, Neil F., 63
Joynt, Robert L., 64
Jurkiewicz, Josh, 37, 80
Jurkiewicz, Maurice J., 80

**K**
Kahn, Eddie, 32
Kaplan, Ernie, 97
Katrana, David J., 108
Kelly, Alexander, 152
Kemper, John, 2–3, 96
Kessering, Ulrich K., 111
Knode, Bob, 71, 77
Knode, Robert E., 77
Koepke, George H., 64
Kresge Research Building, 53
Kusy, R. P., 102
Kuzon, William, 87, 147

**L**
Lampe, Isadore, 28
Lange, Bill, 124
Lange, William, 124
Larsen, Robert, 45–46
Latham, 102
Latham, R. A., 102
Lawrence, Dick, 22
Lawrence, Richard, 115
Lawson, James, 59
Learman, Jeanne, 43
Lee, Denis, 15, 16, 20, 89–90
Lie, Kim, 46
liposuction, 111–112
lip reconstruction, 117
Littler, William, 19
Litton, Clyde, 4
Liverett, David M., 109
Lutz, Lauralee, 14, 15, 17, 35, 37, 64, 65, 132, 137, 141–145, 142, 143
  on Dingman, 132, 134, 163, 168
  on Grabb, 137–138
Lynch, John D., 66
Lyons, Chalmers J., 2

**M**
MacCollum, Malcolm, 76
Manders, Ernie, 40, 48, 84, 126
  Ann Arbor plastic surgery experience, 126, 127
  clinical skin expansion and, 88
  on Dingman, 131–132
  on Grabb, 137

  on Lauralee, 143
  skin flaps and, 62
mandibular ramus of the seventh nerve, 71
Marchac, Daniel, 90
Markley, John M., Jr., 19, 21, 33, 46, 57, 66, 95, 140–141, 148, 152
  clinical microvascular surgery and, 83–84
  hand joint replacement with silicone implants, 74
  hand surgery and, 72–73
  microvascular research, 55–57
  resident rotations and, 43, 47
Marks, Malcolm, 34, 35, 37, 38, 44, 71, 76, 85, 88, 139, 141, 147
  on Grabb, 139
Masters, Frank, 28
Mathes, Stephen J., 80
maxillofacial surgery, 114–116
McClatchey, Ken, 61, 88
McCollum, Biff, 22
McComb, Harold, 102
McCraw, John, 79, 80
  *Atlas of Muscle and Myocutaneous Flaps*, 80
McDowell, Frank, 77–78
McKenny, Peter, 108
McKinney, Peter, 108
McKissock, Paul K., 89
McKissock vertical pedicle technique, 89
Meade, Robert J., 124
Medicaid, 95
Medical Sculpture Service, 16
Medicare, 95
Med Inn, 16
Mes, Louis, 32, 48
  on Dingman, 134
*Message to Garcia, A* (book by Hubbard), 162
metacarpal-phalangeal (MPJ) implants, 74
metatarsal grafts, TMJ reconstruction with, 69–70
Meyer, Rodolphe, 111
Michigan Academy of Plastic Surgery (MAPS)
  history of, 124–125
Michigan State Medical Society, 125
microvascular research, 55–57
Millard, D. Ralph, 9, 97, 98, 101, 139

Millard, Ralph, Jr., 9–10, 98
Milton, Stuart, 78
Mitz, V., 108
Mohs's chemosurgical method, for skin cancer, 75, 76
monkeys, nerve suturing techniques in, 64–65
Morley, George, 86
Morykwas, Michael, 55, 114
Munro, Ian, 31
Musgrave, Ross, 41
Mustarde, J. C., 107, 110
Myers, Bert, 29
    *Skin Flaps*, 77–78, 79
myocutaneous (musculocutaneous) flaps, 79–81
myringotomy, 99

N

Nahai, Foad, 80
nasoendoscopy, 103
naso-orbital fractures, 113
Natvig, Paul, 4, 6–7, 69, 71, 105, 112
    rhinoplasty and, 105
    *Surgery of Facial Fractures*, 70, 112–113
nerve suturing techniques, in monkeys, 64–65
Nesbit, Reed, 68
Neumann, Charles G., 59
Newman, Hack, 33, 34, 64
Newman, M. Haskell, 22, 31–32, 140
    craniofacial surgery and, 117–119
Nguyen, Abram, 108
Nipple reconstruction, 95
Nobel, Gary, 22, 98
Norris, Jim, 63, 82, 130–131, 134, 144
    decubitus ulcers and, 81–82
    on Lauralee, 143
Novark, Bruce, 22, 116, 127, 142
    Ann Arbor plastic surgery experience, 127
    on Grabb, 137
    on Lauralee, 143, 144
    maxillofacial surgery and, 116

O

O'Connor, John, 22
Olesen, Merle, 22
Oneal, Bob, 41, 141
Oneal, Robert M. (RMO), 8–10, 13, 18, 19, 27, 46, 69, 72, 74, 77, 88, 91, 92, 95, 98, 103, 104, 113, 115, 142, 153–154
    and Dingman, 37, 171–173
    eulogy for Grabb, 160
    resident rotations and, 43
orbital capillary hemangioma, 76
Orticochea, Miguel, 79–80, 103
Osler, William, 164–165
otolaryngology, 31
otoplasty, 107

P

palmaris longus graft, 72
Pasyk, Krystyna, 55, 60–62, 71, 76, 88
    "Tissue Expansion: Dividend or Loan?," 62
Pearson, Joseph, 86
Peled, I., 40, 71, 107, 109, 129, 136, 142, 143
    Ann Arbor plastic surgery experience, 129
    on Dingman, 136
    on Lauralee, 143
perfusion takeover, 63
Peyronie, M., 108
Pickrell, K., 92
*Plastic and Reconstructive Surgery (PRS)*, 25, 27, 46, 53, 66
*Plastic Surgery*, 29, 88
*Plastic Surgery—A Concise Guide to Clinical Practice*, 26
*Plastic Surgery in General Surgery Practice*, 28
Plastic Surgery Program, visiting fellows in, 153
Plastic Surgery Section (PSS) Annual Reports, 16, 82, 101
Pollock, Dick, 22
Ponitz, Robert, 71, 115, 142
    maxillofacial surgery and, 114–115
Pool, Robert, 97, 98, 101–102, 152
Posch, Joseph, 45
preserved costal cartilage homografts, 67–68
presurgical palatal orthopedics, 101–102
*Principles and Art of Plastic Surgery, The*, 9–10
prophylactic mastectomy, 93–94
Puckett, C. L., 92

R

Radovan, Chedomir, 59, 87, 88
Radovan Expander, 59, 62

Ralph Millard Society, 121
Ransom, Henry, 15
rat hind limb arterial anastomosis patency model, 57
Rathjen, Art, 89
*Reconstruction and Rehabilitation of the Burned Patient*, 29
reduction mammoplasty, 89–90
Reed O. Dingman Library, 16–17
Reed O. Dingman Society, evolution of, 120–124
Reed, Walter, 30
Rees, Thomas D., 109
Regnault, Paule, 92
Reinisch, John, 78
*Repair and Reconstruction in the Orbital Region*, 110
resident rotations, 39–52
    at Ann Arbor Veterans Administration Hospital, 48–49
    hand rotation, in Detroit, 45–46
    at Saint Joseph Mercy Hospital, 40–44
    teaching conferences, 49–52
    at University of Michigan Hospital, 44–45
    at Wayne County General Hospital, 47
resident selection, 130–131
residents, group images of, 174–183
rhinoplasty, 31, 104–106
Ricker, O. Lee, 66
Rohrich, Rod, 27, 61, 88, 103
    rhinoplasty and, 106
Ron Wexler, Menachem, 63, 68, 95, 109, 117, 128
Rose, Greg, 60
Rosenstein, Sheldon, 95
Rowan, Andrew, 162

S
Saint Joseph Mercy Hospital (SJMH), 5
    Institution of Plastic Surgery Residency Training, 6–10, 150–152
    Joint Commission on Residency Training, 6
    resident rotations at, 40–44
    Section of Plastic Surgery, formation of, 11–22
Sandall, Gary, 71, 76

Sargent, Roland, 53
Sarns, Richard, 99–100
Sasaki, Moto, 154–155
Saturday morning teaching rounds, 50
Schteingart, David, 57
Schulte, Rudy, 87
Seaton, R., 71, 74, 75
secobarbital (Seconal), 43
Seconal (secobarbital), 43
Section of Plastic Surgery (UM Department of Surgery)
    changes in board requirements, and plastic surgery training requirements, 22
    early history of, 13–18
    faculty appointments, 18–21
    formation of, 11–22
    Michigan–Maryland Connection, 21–22
    transitions in, 23–38
Sheen, Jack, 105
Sheflan, Michael, 95
Shields, Sister Mary Xavier, 6, 7
shotgun injuries to the face, 85–86
Silverton, John S., 103
Simons, John, 28
skin cancers, treatment of, 74–76
skin flaps, 29, 62–64, 77–78, 77–79
skin grafting, 28
Skoog, Tord, 108
SMASectomy, 108
Smith, Byron, 31
Smith, David, 146
Smith, Donna, 43
Smith, Ferris, 1, 2, 4, 66
Smith, James W., 26
Smith, Jim, 26, 29
Smith, Lorraine, 73
Smith, William, 84
Southern Michigan State Prison (Jackson Prison)
    resident rotations at, 47–48
Stal, Sam, 106
Steffensen, Wally, 124
Stencil, LuAnn, 43
Stenstrom, Sten J., 107
sternocleidomastoid muscle (SCM), 115
Stevenson, Tom, 37–38, 73, 84
Stilwell, James, 130
Stilwell, Jim, 130
Strauch, Berish, 79
Strombeck, J. O., 89

Strombeck technique, 89
subcutaneous musculo-aponeurotic system (SMAS), 108
*Surgery Clinics of North America*, 68
*Surgery of Facial Fractures*, 70, 112–113

**T**
Tallmadge, G. Kasten, 113
Tamerin, Joseph, 104
Tan, Nick, 76
Tardy, Gene, 105
Taylor, William, 28, 75–76
Teal, Donald F., 93
Tebbets, John, 106
Tessier, P., 34, 117
Thomas, Steve, 60, 62
   "Tissue Expansion: Dividend or Loan?," 62
Thorvaldsson, Sigurdur (Siggy) E., 79, 170
Thursday morning conference, 49–50
Tipton, John, 7, 13, 18, 72
tissue expansion, 57–62
   development of, 57–58
   quality of, 61
"Tissue Expansion: Dividend or Loan?," 62
TMJ reconstruction with metatarsal grafts, 69–70
*Transactions of the American Academy of Ophthalmology*, 68
transaxillary augmentation mammoplasty dissector, 69
transverse island flap, 94
transverse rectus abdominis myocutaneous (TRAM) flap, 94–95
Tuesday afternoon didactic conference, 49
Turcotte, Jeremiah G., 24
Turcotte, Jerry, 84, 146

**U**
unilateral cleft lip (UCL), 96–98
   nose, 102–103
University of Michigan Hospital (UMH)
   Department of Surgery's Section of Plastic Surgery. *See* Section of Plastic Surgery (UM Department of Surgery)
   North Outpatient Building (NOB), 14, 15
   Plastic Surgery Residency Training, 150–152
   research laboratory, 53
   resident rotations at, 44–45
   visiting professors, 149–150

**V**
Valium (diazepam), 43
VanderKolk, Craig, 27, 103
Vasconez, Luis O., 79, 80
Venes, Joan, 119

**W**
Washtenaw County Emergency Medical Technician Training (EMT) program, 29
Watanabe, Mike, 22
Wayne County General Hospital (WCGH)
   resident rotations at, 47
Webster, Richard, 31, 32
weekly Saturday morning research conference, 51
Weiss, Harvey, 41
   on Lauralee, 144–145
Wexler, Ron, 15, 19, 71, 133
   Ann Arbor plastic surgery experience, 128
   craniofacial surgery and, 118
   face-lifting and, 109
   lip reconstruction and, 117
   McKissock vertical pedicle technique, 89
   skin flaps and, 63
White, Tim, 56
Wilensky, Bob, 22, 41, 71, 77
   on Dingman, 135
Wilensky, Robert, 41, 77, 93, 133
William Grabb Lectureship, 123
Winkler, James M., 69
Winkler, Jim, 69, 71
Wisenthall, Larry, 63
Woodburn, Russell, 71
Work, Walter, 12, 27

**X**
Xanax (alprazolam), 43

**Z**
Z-plasty, 27, 66, 68, 69, 100, 108

www.ingramcontent.com/pod-product-compliance
Lightning Source LLC
Chambersburg PA
CBHW050525170426
43201CB00013B/2085